CW00408993

Fit For a Bride

by Greg Doyle CPT-ACSM

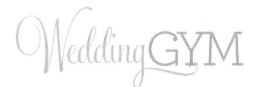

This book is for every bride out there who wants to look beautiful in their dress on their wedding day. My goal is to help you lose weight, sculpt and tone your entire body, so you are happy with yourself on the inside and out!
Now Let's Get Going!

Contents

How the step-by-step plan designed by NYC celebrity trainer, Greg Doyle, will get you in the best shape of your life for your wedding!

Get started with Week 1 of the step-by-step system.

Your Initial Consult. See exactly what you'll need to get and do, for your total body transformation.

See how superfoods will help you cleanse and shed the pounds to rebuild a slimmer, sexier, healthier you!

Full body bridal workouts with the right exercises to boost your metabolism, burn calories, and sculpt your new bridal body!

See why rest is crucial to looking more beautiful, healthier, and slimmer.

A quick summary of the 4 Step Plan to your new bridal body.

- Customizing the 4 Step Plan for your body

- *Fit For a Bride* Dos and Don'ts

- How to boost your fat loss even faster

- And MORE!

Super delicious recipes for those who want to get creative. Most only take a few minutes to prepare!

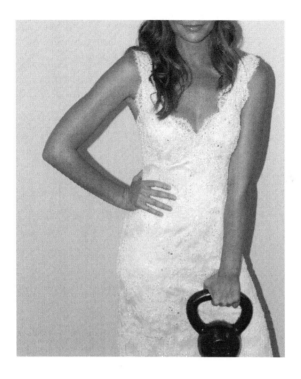

Intro: *Fit For a Bride* 4-Step Plan

First off, congrats on the engagement! You've beaten the odds and found that special someone and that's no easy task in today's world.

Next, I'd like to thank you for purchasing this book! You are holding in your hands one of the most effective plans ever created to help brides-to-be, like you, shed fat and tone up so you look amazing in your dress (and the hundreds, if not thousands of pictures) on perhaps the most special day of your life. You will discover things in this book that you won't find anywhere else;

secrets that expose the myths that are keeping you from losing weight.

My job is to transform your body. I will show you EXACTLY what you need to eat and do in order to completely transform your body, leaving you lean and slimmer than ever, by your wedding. Best part is, I've taken everything you need and created a step-by-step system so you can lose weight, even if you've struggled in the past!

This book will get you SEXY AS ALL HECK!

Listen, I've been doing this for a while; it's what I love to do. My clients have always reached success through a path not of discipline, but of encouragement and support in their fitness goals. For me, it's a win-win situation. It doesn't get better than that. I take brides-to-be and unleash a completely new body for them. Everyone is a masterpiece, and everyone (you included) has that potential ability to sculpt and shape that masterpiece body for all to see. With the specific nutritional plan and certain exercise programs included in this book, I use proven science combined with my years of proven experience to help you slim down, flatten your stomach, and tone up every inch of your body so you look stunning in your wedding dress.

All eyes on you:

You'll get the same tools I use with my clients to create a body that maybe you never thought was possible. A body that you'll proudly showcase walking down the aisle, as everyone you love watches you on the happiest day of your life. Let's face it, your wedding is a party, a big party, and you are the spotlight of that party. Everyone will be watching you, you've hired a photographer and/or videographer to document the entire affair and you want to look damn good.

I know for so many women that after the excitement of the engagement passes, the next thought is: "Oh crap, I better look freakin' amazing in my dress!" And why shouldn't you? It's your day, and you want to look more than good, you want to look *gooooood*. I also know that many brides turn to not-so-safe diets, "fat burning" pills, or other drastic measures to lose the weight in ways that are less than healthy and even less effective.

If you're like most women who have turned to these "quick fix" methods in the past, you know they rarely work. I'll share with you what DOES work.

In this book, I'll show you the 4 Step method I've been using for years to get the perfect bridal body for my clients in half the time! Forget about counting calories, starving yourself, or giving up your favorite foods. With *Fit For a Bride,* I'm revealing my step-by-step process in detail, so you are able to easily shed the pounds and sculpt that sexy body while staying healthy and sane!

Fit For a Bride 4-Step Plan:

1) Assess for Your Dress: Set your goals and get real motivation!

2) Eat Your Way Skinny: Eat more and burn more. Discover the right foods that slim and satisfy!

3) Sculpt and Shed: The workouts you should be doing, but aren't…All in UNDER 30 minutes!

4) Recover and Reassess: How to rest your way to a younger, healthier and sexier you!

Using these 4 steps, you discover everything you need to get rid of that extra fat and tone those stubborn trouble areas in only 12 weeks.

You will never have to give up any foods, and you won't have to count calories! (I'll explain why it's counterproductive later.) We are going to use some super effective techniques that will create a slimmer and sexier you from the inside out.

I'll show you why you should:

- Never count another calorie!

- Eat carbs. You don't have to give up carbs to lose weight!

- Eat real and delicious "superfoods" to boost health *and* fat loss.

- Never give up your favorite foods!

I'm also going to show you simple 30 minute workouts to get your metabolism rocking on full throttle again, so you are burning more calories 24/7, sculpting a sexy bridal body, and while perfecting your posture. (You DON'T want to be a Hunchback Bride do you?)

In short, you are going to get you sexy and slim, and have fun doing it.

You've been lied to when it comes to weight loss:

Diets alone don't work. The sad truth is that **most people (90%) who start a diet will fail and regain all the weight they lost, plus more, within one year,** and exercise alone is not enough to change your body. (Trust me, I'm a personal trainer and even I'll admit that exercise alone is not the key to transforming your body).

The good news? Using slimming superfoods found in our meal plans, you don't need to diet. Combining this with the super effective fat crushing workouts, you'll be able to achieve a body that you never thought was possible.

But is it really for you?

If you basically want to look sexier than ever on your wedding night and beyond, then this is the book for you. If you tried diet after diet in the past only to be left hungrier, heavier, and just frustrated and depressed, then this book is for you. Are you exercising all the time, seeing no results, and wondering what you're doing wrong? Then, yep you guessed it, this book is for you. If you want to eat delicious foods for every meal while losing weight and burning fat, then again, this book is probably for you.

If you are looking to lose 40 lbs. this weekend, then maybe this book isn't for you. If you'd rather cheat your body and your health by resorting to some "quick fix" strategies found in pill bottles, then perhaps you're not cut out for this system. I will tell you that any of those "lose 20 lbs. OVERNIGHT" products will not give you the body you want and deserve, and you most certainly won't be able to maintain those "results". (So good luck in that bikini on your honeymoon...)

I'm not saying this to be mean, but to be realistic. If those pills/powders/whatevers did work, then close to 70% of America still wouldn't be overweight, would they? I will tell you that if you incorporate the easy meal plans and the quick workouts into your daily routine, you'll be getting results like never before, it's that simple. **And these are results that will LAST, you won't be losing water weight, you'll be losing FAT, burning it off and keeping it off!**

What you do now is making you fat...

As a top NYC trainer, I have clients who need results - plain and simple. If I had them doing what 99% of people are doing in the gym, they would get nowhere and I'd be out of a job. Fortunately, I know my stuff. I get results, and I'm willing to share these personal training insider secrets with you in this book. I'll show you where you're going wrong, what works, and then spell out the workouts plans to tone and sculpt your new body week by week.

Listen, if you knew exactly what to eat/do, and were doing it, well...you wouldn't need this book. But let's face it, with the media and other "fitness experts" constantly telling you about this or that new "diet", I wouldn't blame you if you were unsure of what to actually do. Unless you do countless hours of research (lucky for you, I happen to love that), then there's no doubt you'd be confused on what "new food" or exercise to use to lose weight and shape up. Heck, I would be.

There's also no doubt that some of the things you are doing, and the foods you are eating are actually making you gain or re-tain your fat. In fact, most people don't realize that some of the foods they thought were "healthy" are actually causing them to gain weight!

I'm going to make things simple and take you step-by-step to the body of your dreams for your wedding. I've even included some supercharged tips to help you fast track your fat loss in case you have less than 12 weeks until your wedding, or just want more results in less time!

The guide to the slim and sexy bride - How it was born:

When I tell people what I do, they often look at me like I'm crazy. "You train brides?!" This is usually followed by, "Wow, you must deal with a lot of bridezillas huh?" I tell them that I love what I do, that out of all my clients, the brides were always my most favorite to work with. That's why I started a company devoted to real fitness and healthy fat loss for brides. Some people think I'm crazy, but what they don't realize is that I'm able to help brides feel great about their bodies, but also about themselves. That's powerful. So I how did I get here and how did this book even come into existence?

Who am I and why I'm doing this?

A little about me, as a personal trainer in NYC, I love fitness, and I love food. In fact the reason I got into fitness was because I loved food a little too much.

See, I wasn't born a fitness freak, or skinny, or physically gifted. I was a chubby kid, who wasn't that good at sports. I thought Twinkies, powdered donuts, and Yoo-hoos were a well-rounded breakfast. But I was able to turn myself around using exercise and food to get leaner and stronger, physically and mentally.

I was a chunker.

As a child, I grew up with a pretty big sweet tooth, and I was a chunker. I wasn't obese, but I was chubby (my mom called me "husky", thanks ma), and my friends called me "Fat Greg". I played it off, and became the class clown where I was still relatively popular. I had a lot of friends, but I'd be lying if I said it didn't bother me. When I was in 8th grade, I'd had enough and wanted a change. For Christmas that year I got a home gym, the kind Chuck Norris advertised on TV. It was the best Christmas ever.

I read every health and fitness magazine I could find and taught myself how to be fit, and eat better. By the end of 8th grade I wasn't a chunker anymore. I then decided to join the freshman football team going into high school. I was awful at football, but loved working out in the weight room.

Soon I had a six-pack for the first time, and my friends would come to me when they had questions about exercise or nutrition. It felt great, and I loved how I was able to transform myself. Heading to college, I quickly realized I wanted to study exercise and nutrition, and did so at the University of Delaware.

After I graduated, I applied to several personal training companies in NYC. I quickly found somewhere where I had the chance to work privately one-on-one with clients who, let's just say, were the top clientele in NYC. I did it all, and I was good at what I did. I worked with hedge fund managers, billionaires, world famous artists, movie stars, and even royalty, but at the end of the day, the brides-to-be were my favorites!

Working with brides:

Training brides is always exciting, because I get to work with motivated individuals getting them ready for their big day. They are anxious and excited, and I always love the challenge of getting my clients to their goals by a deadline.

After their weddings, my clients usually say, "People kept coming up and telling me how amazing I looked, or how defined my arms looked". Or they tell me that I had no idea how much the workouts helped them to de-stress in some of the most stressful weeks of their lives. I have to admit, it makes me feel awesome.

Realizing that I want to reach more than just the handful of brides I train privately in NYC, I got a suggestion from a client that I write a book. I took up the challenge and wrote what you're holding in your hands now. Knowing that there is so much misinformation out there, I wanted brides all across the world to be able to get the truth and use what works. Modeling this book after my online weight loss coaching program, I've put together everything needed to lose fat and tone up, step-by-step right here in this book.

The *Fit For a Bride* plan - how it will work for you:

While this book will show you the steps to fat loss simplicity, I still need one thing from you if you want to transform your body into that leaner, healthier version of you. You NEED to take action. This book spells out what to do to get in super "wedding" shape. It's a compilation of years of hands-on bridal training, research, and experience, but if you do not use it (I don't care how many times you read it) you will get **nowhere.** That leaves a frumpier, heavier you standing at the alter wondering, "Did I do everything I could have?" but already knowing the answer.

DO NOT LET THAT BE YOU.

I spent countless hours researching and writing to put this book together, and I did it, because I know the secret to losing fat and keeping it off. I want you to know it too! To me, it's unfair to keep it stuck in my oddly shaped head, so here it is, **but you HAVE to USE IT!**

You are going to take action, because you want to look amazing when all eyes are on you. You want your 6 yr. old grandchildren to look at your wedding day photographs one day and ask you, "Hey Grand mammy, WHO'S that sexy chica in that picture"? And with a smile and a twinkle in your eyes, you'll say, **"That was me grandchild, that sexy chica was me".** So let's do this. The power is yours, it always has been, I'm here to guide you and show you what to do.

Are you ready for it?

Ah that's a dumb question, of course you are, now let's go!

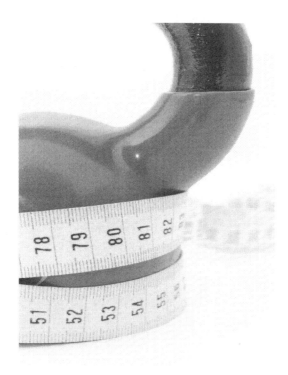

Getting Started:
Fit For a Bride Prepping

You've stuck around and decided you want to look better than you ever have before, and because you're still reading this, it means you're one of only a small percentage of people whom take action and get what they want. CONGRATS!

Now let's get right into it.

What this book will do for you

Get ready to look slimmer, younger, and more toned. The meal plans and workouts will leave you with more energy, better skin and hair, standing taller and more elegant with perfect posture, and create a new you by the end of the 12 weeks.

The Plan

This book has meal plans and workouts that have been designed to last for 12 weeks. This is usually the optimal amount of time to make a real and very noticeable change in one's body and appearance. With that being said, you might have more weight to lose at the end of the 12 weeks. The great part about this system is it can be tailored to your needs. Shorten it, or keep going with it if you find that you want to lose even more after the 12 weeks. Many brides have found that they continue with the meals and workouts even after the wedding, because they love their sexier new bodies.

The 4 Steps Breakdown

For the 4 Step plan we want to keep it as simple as possible. Below are the main steps to your new bridal body. The book moves step-by-step with each chapter, including all the details for you to rock this! By reading through and following steps, you will finally get the results you deserve, and a body you will be amazed with.

• Step 1: Assess for Your Dress

Like with any client I have, the first thing to do is assess where you are now, so you can get to where you want to be. For the first week, you will write down your goal, so you know exactly what you want, and when you want to achieve it by. Every Friday, you will weigh in and take a full body picture. This keeps you accountable to yourself, and lets you know if you're melting the fat, or need to turn it up a bit. You will also perform a workout assessment each month in order to see if you are getting leaner AND fitter. Once you've finished the assessments in week 1, you'll move on to Step 2.

Step 2: Eat Your Way Skinny

For the meal plans, we keep it simple and delicious. You eat 3 meals a day, with an optional snack. All the meals use superfoods to keep you full and, because it's real food, not processed fake stuff. You will be eating much healthier. You will cycle through days of higher and lower carbohydrates, so there is no giving up carbs completely, but you still lose weight quickly. Each week has a cheat meal included, so as long as you are eating according to the plan, you get to eat whatever you want 1 day each week. This keeps you sane and keeps your metabolism rocking hard. I'll also explain what drinks you want include, and which ones you'll want to avoid.

Looking at the 12 weeks of meal plans you will realize we included lots of meals. Many brides interchange and swap meals from different days, which is fine. You will probably find a few meals that you really like and end up sticking to them. That's OK too! When you think about it, most people eat the same things day in and day out anyways, but I figured having some more options is always fun.

Step 3: Total Body Sculpting

In Step 3, I'll introduce the most effective exercises and workouts designed to sculpt and tone your entire body while melting the fat. To save you time, I've created 30 minute or less workouts that are super effective and tailored to your bridal body. These will be short, but intense workouts to challenge you and transform your body. For even better results, I'll show you the cardio you should be doing in-between the workouts if you want faster fat loss. You will see how to get results that will make others envious, and why not? This is *your* big day.

• Step 4: Rest & Reassess

For an ultimately lean and healthy bridal body, getting more sleep is critical. I will show you tips to increase the amount and quality of sleep you get so you look all the more slim and toned for it. Reassessments are done weekly so you can make adjustments if you are not exactly on track. You'll also find out how sex can help in the quest to get lean and healthy.

PREPPING:

Kitchen Makeover

As you get ready to start the 4 Step Plan, one of the first things to do is a kitchen makeover. If you are serious about really changing your body, then your environment needs to change. This means removing any foods that will sabotage your new lean body.

There is a law that states:

**"If you have something in your kitchen,
you will eventually eat it."**

It also works the other way:

**"If you DON'T have something in your kitchen,
you can't eat it."**

This is why I included the Kitchen Makeover Guide in Chapter 6, and right under that, the Grocery Lists to get you started. If you want to seriously lose weight and shed fat, understand that you can't eat healthy if you don't have healthy foods.

We've all been there before. A stressful day at work, you were so busy that you skipped lunch, and now that you're home, that Nutella looks so good. You take a spoonful, and before you know it, you've finished the WHOLE thing. Bam, that just wiped out a weeks' worth of eating well and busting your butt in the gym. Not worth it. While it may be something you can treat yourself to on cheat days, it can't be there all the time, or at work either.

What You'll Need to Get for the Plan

Here are some of the things that will make your weight loss so much easier. Most of these things you can find online, Amazon. com is a great place to find these (No I don't get paid by them, it's just a great one stop shopping site, and I do buy all my stuff through them).

Below, I've only included those things I know are of quality and are affordable.

For the meals:

- **Food:** I know this seems obvious, but you'll have to go shopping to have the healthy food to eat!

- **Blender:** Great for smoothies and making your own sauces. I have an Oster brand blender that I got for $20, and I use it every day. No need to go super expensive!

- **Non-Stick Frying Pan:** If you don't have one, get one. I use one of these 2-3 times a day to make quick eggs or chicken.

- **Blender Bottle:** These little BPA-free plastic shaker bottles are awesome to store a smoothie for on-the-go eating. They won't open up in your bag. Go for the 28 oz. size.

- **Tupperware Containers:** Use these to store precooked foods for easy lunches Ziploc bags are key as well for throwing a handful of nuts in for a snack on the go.

For the workouts:

- **Body Fat Scale:** (Not necessary but recommended) Many companies are making affordable weighing scales that also measure your body fat levels. While weighing is great, it's just one way to measure your success and having body fat % measurements is even better.

- **Kettlebell:** You can find these online (I get mine on Amazon.com) or you can go to your local sporting goods store. Beginners should go with a 20-25 lb. kettlebell. More experienced exercisers should look for 25-30 lb. kettlebells.

- **Medicine Ball:** Look for these at local sporting goods stores or online, from 6-8lbs for a beginner, intermediate exercisers should go for 8-10 lb. weight.

- **Jump Rope:** My favorite rope that I use with my clients is the Valero speed rope. You can find these for around $8 on Amazon.com, and are one of the best pieces of fitness equipment you can buy for your money.

- **Resistance Band:** For most exercisers, you'll want to use a medium resistance band with handles.

- **Yoga Mat:** For exercises on the floor, yoga mats are great to have. You can pick these up at any sporting goods store or online. Most brands will work fine, and you can find them for under $ 10 to 20.

Lose Weight Right NOW:

There is something that I have my clients try out after their first consult, and it's something that leads to weight loss almost immediately, even if you don't change your diet or start exercising. If you want to know how to start this today, then let's move on to the next chapter!

Remember:

The next 12 weeks are going to pass by regardless of what you do, or don't do. So what do you want to look like in 12 weeks?

Chapter One

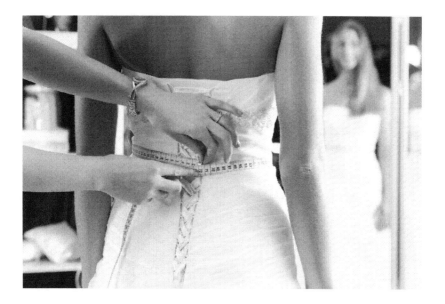

STEP 1: Assess For Your Dress

It's your wedding day and you're standing in your dress. You've been waiting for this day forever and planning for it even longer. Looking in the mirror you see the dress fits perfectly. You look stunning, and because you know you look so good, there is no doubt you are going to enjoy every minute of that day (and the photos afterwards.)

That's the goal. The goal isn't to drop 5 or 10 lbs, but to look your best and have an amazing day that will never be forgotten. But before you get there, we're going to have to start somewhere, and that somewhere is here and now.

In Step 1, Week 1 is the assessment of your dress. It's the start of the program and defines where and who you want to be on your wedding day. Do you want to be the bride who has trouble fitting into her dress on the big day? Or the bride who has to have her dress taken in, because you've slimmed all over? It's up to you.

Now let's set some solid goals, do a few assessments to get started, and create a place to start from so goals can be measured to show your progress. Together, we will meet your goals.

Week 1, Part 1 - Challenge

Before we get into the goals, I want to give you a challenge for the week. You might just find that you're lighter by the end of the next 7 days, without changing your diet or exercise!

Lose weight NOW - Secrets to immediate weight loss

One of my clients (I'll call her "Anne" for the book), came back to me after 2 weeks of her initial consult to start training. She had lost 9 lbs. since our first meeting. I asked her, "What did you do?" I wanted to know if Anne was eating differently or exercising more. She replied, "No, I didn't really change anything, except that I listened to what you told me about eating when I was hungry. I was amazed at how many times I was eating just to eat! I wasn't hungry at all when I was eating before and was totally unaware of it, so I just ate when I was hungry and didn't eat when I wasn't hungry like you told me."

Anne was shocked at how such a seemingly simple statement could provide such dramatic results. I'll add that she wasn't eating healthier, she wasn't exercising more, she was merely listening to her body for once. I wasn't shocked at all.

I know that this is one of the most powerful tools I use with my clients, which will be the foundation for your fat loss if you follow it.

"Eat when you are hungry and do not eat when you are not hungry"

I'm not sure if one sentence has had more of an impact on my clients' fat loss than this one right here. **Now STOP and read it again.** I'm serious. I know, because it's so simple sounding that it might be easy to just pass over it and think, "OK Greg, everyone knows this, duh!" But does everyone follow this? NO! If you are at a healthy weight, you are the minority in the US. That's scary to me. Anyways, READ the statement above again!

Tattoo this on your face. Write it on your hands, your wall, your fridge, put it as the background of your phone. Keep it somewhere you will see it every day. (Don't tattoo it on your face...).*

"Eat when you are hungry and do not eat when you are not hungry"

Why it works

You are a walking calorie absorber.

Humans evolved to store calories, plain and simple. If our ancestors didn't become master calorie storers, they would have died off when there was any type of food shortage. (There were no supermarkets around 100,000 years ago, and definitely no Dunkin Donuts.) This was OK, because we moved around, working, gathering, and hunting. We usually had just enough food to get by.

Flash forward to today. Most of us don't hunt or gather. We sit for more than 75% of the day and have an ever-ready flow of food at all times. It's safe to bet that you could probably find a meal within 10 minutes at any point throughout the day. It should be no wonder so many of us are fat. Our bodies are just doing their jobs, and doing it well!

According to the CDC, **nearly 70% of the US is now over-weight/obese**. People say it's sugar, it's high fructose syrup, it's saturated fat, it's carbs, it's salt, it's processed foods, it's etc., etc., etc., yet there's another obvious answer. Now yes, of course we need to cut out processed foods, no doubt, but if you look back to the upper class of European society in the 1600s and 1700s, they were FAT with no GMOs, non-organic foods, or high fructose syrup.

They ate more and were larger, because of it. It showed that they had money and could afford lots of food. Don't be like them.

The ever expanding gas tank

If your car's gas tank was full, would you go and keep putting more gas into it? No, yet we do this every day to ourselves when we eat and are not hungry. Except, our bodies can keep expanding and stores that food as fat. Around your thighs, stomach, hips, and arms.

The problem is that **it takes roughly 20 minutes after the stomach is already full for the signals to reach the brain to tell you that you are full.** That gives you 20 minutes to continue stuffing an already full stomach, especially if you eat too fast…

Your challenge:

For the next 7 days, before you go to eat anything, ask yourself this question:

"Am I actually hungry right now?"

Now, I'm not talking about having an appetite after you've seen a cupcake, I'm talking a legit feeling of hunger. It's a "Yes" or "No" answer.

Write down or record this for the next week. At each meal, indicate whether or not you were hungry when you reached for food. You can write it down on paper or make a note on your phone. By doing this for the next week, you will become aware of how you eat and will create new habits leading to a slimmer and leaner body in no time.

If you decide to continue after the 7 days, you certainly can (a lot of my successful clients continue to do this every day.)

5 top tips to losing weight NOW (without dieting)

1. **Eat when you are hungry:** By listening to your body, you can put a stop to the mindless munching that has caused most Americans to gain weight like crazy.

2. **Slow down:** Try enjoying your food for once. Most people rush through their meals. Slow it down and actually ENJOY eating. You'll be amazed at how quickly you feel full.

3. **Stop eating crap:** Honestly, life's too short to fill up on calories that never tasted amazing in the first place. Can you even recall half the food you ate last week? Chances are it was mediocre at best and not deserving of being stored as fat in your body.

4. **Chew your food:** This seems obvious, but next time you eat, pay attention to the food you are eating and chew it all the way through. You'd be amazed how many people ba-

sically swallow their food in a rush, and then wonder why they have digestion issues. Food is to be enjoyed.

5. **Sit down and eat:** We live in an eat-on-the-go society and by rushing through meals, it's going to be tough (if not impossible) to follow the 4 tips above. Take at least 30 minutes to eat your next meal.

And Remember:

"Eat when you are hungry and do not eat when you are not hungry"

Week 1, Part 2 - Getting Sexy with Goals

The next part of Week 1 is to set up another goal to move towards for the next 12 weeks. I know it sounds cliché, but you need goals to get anywhere you want to be. Without goals, you'll never know if you are getting closer or further away from that slimmer, leaner, and sexier new you.

5 steps to goal setting for a sexier you!

1) Pick a goal (DON'T be realistic…Aim HIGH)

The first step is to choose a goal. Have you always wanted to lose those 10, 20, or even 50 lbs.? Shoot for it. Aim high - be a little unrealistic. People have the tendency to aim low, because it's what they expect. They don't expect to lose 30 pounds, because they've never done it before, so they say, "I wanna lose 10 lbs.!" What a way to dream big. Instead, aim for that 30 lbs. Heck, the worst that can happen is you fall short and lose 20 lbs., when the most you've ever lost was 10!

Examples of common wedding goals:

* Fit into a certain dress size.

* Losing X amount of pounds.

* Fitting into that certain pair of jeans or outfit that you love, which has gotten a little tight recently.

* Seeing definition in the arms, back, and stomach.

* Lowering body fat % to a certain number.

2) Know WHY you are reaching for that goal. (Have a powerful WHY behind it)

You need to want it bad. Maybe you want to lose 25lbs, because that's what you weighed in high school or college. It was the slimmest you ever were, and you want to show off a little bit to those who haven't seen you in years. Maybe you just want to show up your sister-in-law. Who knows? You want to look your best and prove people wrong. **HAVE A STRONG ENOUGH WHY**, otherwise change your goal until it's a strong enough motivator.

3) Imagine yourself already there.

Your daily habits determine who you become. When you start to imagine you are already that slimmer and leaner version of yourself, and really believe you are that new healthy person, you'll start to act the way that leaner slimmer you would act.

Start thinking, **"What would Slimmer/Leaner/Healthier/ Lighter (YOUR NAME) Do?"** Would "Slimmer Me" skip this workout? Probably not. Would "Leaner Me" prepare food so that she has delicious and quick healthy meals all week? Probably.

Would 15 lbs. lighter make me spend an hour on Facebook and then say there is no time for a workout? Probably not.

What habits does the slimmer/leaner/sexier you have?

4) Have a plan to get there.

If you want to drive from NYC to LA, getting in the car with no map or GPS doesn't make sense. You'll get lost and end up in Canada, or maybe West Virginia.

If you desperately want to lose weight, but have no plan, I don't care how bad you want it, you won't get it. Thankfully, you now have in your hands the exact plan to your new sexier self!

5) Tell someone your goal… GET ACCOUNTABLE!!!

If you weren't serious about having a crazy nice body for your wedding, then you wouldn't have bought this book. You wouldn't have read up to this page. This is a serious endeavor, so let's get serious about staying committed, and nothing says "I'm committed" like sharing your goals with friends and family. These are the people who will help keep you on track, because you NEED outside support.

Get it now, and you'll be more motivated to stay consistent. You'll get better results, lose more fat, and look more toned. You'll thank me, I promise.

Below, write in your goals. Include the "why" behind it, "what" would happen if you reached this goal, as well as what would happen if you didn't reach this goal. If you have the electronic version of this book, you'll need to get a piece of paper and write it out there. Either way, write it down and then keep it somewhere you'll see it every day.

I Am Going To: _____

_____

_____

____ by this date: _____

I WANT this because: _____

_____

_____

_____

What healthy habits does the "Slimmer/Leaner/Sexier Me" have (LIST THEM):

*

*

*

*

OK GREAT! Seriously, don't pass by this chapter without really thinking about what you want and writing it down somewhere. It's going to be this motivation that will help you succeed, as it has helped my clients succeed.

Without a goal and a plan, you are just going to be driving around aimlessly, all while you have somewhere important to get to.....YOUR WEDDING!

Week 1, Part 3 - Assessments

OK, so we just set goals, now this is how to measure whether you're getting closer to them each week. You'll start with some easy initial assessments, then you'll have weekly and monthly assessments. Here's where to start:

Initial (Week 1): To start, we will need some baseline info, but we'll keep it simple. Take a "before" picture and your weight on Day 5, or Friday of Week 1. You'll then perform a workout assessment or "Test Day" on the same day.

Weekly (Every Friday): Every Friday, you'll record your weight and take a full body picture. This allows you to not only see your weight change each week, but also get a visual feedback. Don't worry, no one will see these. I also strongly suggest you measure body fat percent if you can as well.

Monthly (Every 30 Days): Every 30 days, you will see that on Friday, "Test Day" is found instead of the workout. You'll perform this same fitness test that you first performed in the initial "Test Day". You'll be amazed to see that not only will you get slimmer and more toned, but you'll be more athletic too!

(For a free downloadable monthly calendar with easy to follow assessment reminders and workouts, go to www.weddinggym.com/bookextras and get yours todays.)

***Notes About Weight:** Because the scale weighs everything (fat, bones, muscle tissue, organs), it can only give you a general idea of what is going on in the body and shouldn't be used alone when trying to track your wedding weight loss success. This is one reason why we need to use pictures and body fat measurements when possible.

Taking your "Before" picture

In order to actually see your transformation, you'll want to take pictures each week. By showing as much skin as possible, you'll be able to see real changes. To keep things consistent, take the pictures and weigh yourself at the SAME time every week. Body weight fluctuates throughout the day, so taking it in the morning one week and in the afternoon the next week would give you inaccurate numbers. I recommend doing it in the morning before breakfast. Get the full body, including the side and back for the best visuals. Remember, that although you won't see crazy differences between each week, after only a few weeks, you'll start to see a slimmer you.

Record your weight here

week 1

week 2

week 3

week 4

week 5

week 6

week 7

week 8

week 9

week 10

week 11

week 12

Fitness Assessments:
Are you *Fit For a Bride?*

"Test Day" fitness assessments
and how to do them

Below you'll find the "Test Day" fitness tests. These are fitness tests, like jumping rope or burpees that will give you a snapshot of your current state of fitness. You'll be able to see how you improve in getting stronger and building endurance as you get leaner and more toned week by week. You'll need a stopwatch or use your phone, if it has a stopwatch setting, for the timed exercises.

How to do the Assessments:

Below is the fitness assessment that you'll do on Day 5, Day 30, Day 60, and Day 90.

- You'll move from one exercise to the next and rest when there is a rest indicated.

- Record your results in the table below.

- Below are the exercises and how many reps or time you'll do the exercise for. Really push it here. You want to be getting in every rep you can, while maintaining proper form.

- Give 100% EVERY single time. If you don't go all out for these tests, you'll never be able to see how much you've progressed throughout the 12 weeks.

- Check out www.weddinggym.com/bookextras for a video showing how to do all the exercises below!

TEST DAY workout

#1 Kettlebell Swings:

The Movement: Stand holding a kettlebell in front of you, with your feet slightly wider than shoulder width. Keep a slight bend in the knees as you bend your butt back behind you, keeping your back straight. Your back shouldn't round over, watch yourself in the mirror if you need to. Forcefully pop your hips forward, thrusting your hips straight ahead. This should start to swing the kettlebell forward. Keep driving the butt backwards, thrusting forward as the kettlebell swings higher and higher up to your head level. Your arms shouldn't be lifting, just holding on to the kettlebell as your hips do all the work.

How Many: As many as you can you do in 30 seconds with proper form.

(Use a Medicine Ball Scoop if you need to.)

RESULTS:

Day 5: _____

Day 30: _____

Day 60: _____

Day 90: _____

REST 1 Minute then move onto Pushups

#2 Pushups:

The Movement: While lying face down on the floor, hands and feet should be shoulder width apart. Contract your stomach and push your body up using your hands. Try to keep your elbows close to your body as you come up, and avoid letting your hips sag down. Imagine your body is a solid piece of wood as it rises up off the ground.

How Many: As many reps as you can do in 1 minute.

(If you cannot perform regular push ups, drop to knees and start there.)

RESULTS:

Day 5: _____

Day 30:_____

Day 60: _____

Day 90:_____

REST- 3-5 Minutes then move on to Jump Squats

#3 Jump Squats:

The Movement: Start with feet shoulder width apart, arms raised above your head. Squat down by lowering your hips back and bending at the knees (as if you were bending back to sit on a bench behind you), while also swinging the arms down until your thighs are parallel with the floor, then jump up, swinging the arms up with you. Land back down into the squat position and continue.

How Many: As many reps as you can do in 30 seconds.

RESULTS:

Day 5: _____

Day 30:_____

Day 60: _____

Day 90:_____

REST 1 Minute then move on to Plank

#4 Plank:

The Movement: Get into a push up position, but with your forearms resting on the ground, supporting your upper body. Only your forearms and feet should touch the ground. Keep your back parallel with the floor, making sure your hips don't sag. Keep your stomach braced as if you were getting ready for someone to punch you in the stomach.

How Many: Hold for as many seconds as possible.

(Perform on forearms; if you can't do forearms, perform in a push up position.)

RESULTS:

Day 5: _____

Day 30:_____

Day 60:_____

Day 90:_____

REST 1 Minute then move onto Jump Rope

#5 Jump Rope:

The Movement: Hop on both feet while using your wrists to swing the jump rope. Once you hear the rope hit the floor, get ready to jump. If you have serious jump rope issues, just drop down the rope and do just the jumping, or what I call "Imaginary Jump Rope."

How Many: For this final test, you are going to push as hard as you can. Jump rope for as long as you can, until failure. (Meaning, you really can't skip another skip, legs are fatigued, and you feel that burn in the calf muscles.)

RESULTS

Day 5: _____

Day 30: _____

Day 60: _____

Day 90: _____

FINISHED! Make sure you recorded your results for each exercise and then give yourself a huge pat on the back!

Notes:

- **Reps or repetitions:** The completion of the given exercise, for example, for a squat bending down and then standing back straight up would be 1 rep or repetition.

- **AMRAP: As Many Reps As Possible.** If it says 30 Seconds AMRAP, you would perform as many reps as you could in under 30 seconds.

For Video on how to do the Test Day assessment workout, go to www.weddinggym.com/bookextras for more guidance on EXACTLY how to do each exercise.

Week 1 Summary & Checklist

✓ Setting Goals (Monday)

✓ Initial weigh in (Monday)

✓ Getting things you'll need (Tuesday)

✓ Are you Really Hungry? Yes or No (Monday-Sunday)

✓ Kitchen makeover & grocery shopping (Wednesday)

✓ Take "Before" picture (Friday)

✓ Fitness assessment "Test Day" (Friday)

✓ Try out recipes from meal plan (Monday-Sunday)

FAQ for Week 1

What about meals and workouts during Week 1?

- **Meals:** As for the meal plans, you are not required to stick to any certain meals at all. The actual meal plans won't start until Week 2. You can and *should* check out some of the meals from the meal plans, and some of the recipes at the end of the book!

Make sure to hydrate as well, general rule: ½ your bodyweight in ounces per day.

- **Workouts:** You won't be starting any workouts until Week 2, but you will see there is a "Test Day" on Friday of Week 1. This is a workout assessment that will test your level of fitness and create a baseline to see where you are physically so you can improve over the next few weeks!

(While the workouts don't officially start until Monday on Week 2, you can get in some cardio and start practicing some of the resistance exercises that are found in the workouts.)

What to do after Week 1?

Once you complete Week 1, you will then start with the meal plans and workouts provided week by week starting with Week 2, and moving on each week to the next week's set of meal plans and workouts. The total 12 weeks are broken down into 3 phases, each phase basically being 4 weeks, or 1 month, in total.

Every Friday you will take the pictures and weight, (and body fat % if possible) while recording the amount of reps you perform each week during the workouts so that you can push it the next week.

Use the grocery lists found in Chapter 6 to give you a good idea of what you'll need to pick up each week at the store. If you decide to customize the meal plans to you, then make sure you buy the foods you'll need for each week.

Remember: No one just wakes up fat, or wakes up skinny. Week after week of rocking the meal plans and workouts will add up and before you know it, you'll be a new you, but ONLY if you stick it out.

Oh, and …

EAT ONLY WHEN YOU ARE HUNGRY,

DO NOT EAT WHEN YOU ARE NOT HUNGRY.

Now let's move on to one of my most favorite subjects in the world…. FOOD.

I'll show you what food myths have been keeping you fat, real delicious food I used to get accelerated results with my bridal clients, and how you can start to get them too!

Chapter Two

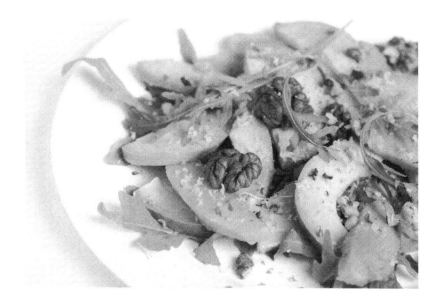

STEP 2: Eat Your Way Skinny

I'm going to be blunt and honest with you here. You've come to me for help, and I'm going to give you the advice I would give to my clients and close friends.

The fact is you can bust your butt in the gym all day every day and still get nowhere if your nutrition is not great. You may not want to hear this, but it's a fact. And unless you start getting serious about what you eat everyday, you'll be wasting your time and money and energy at the gym.

Why would a personal trainer admit that? Because it's the truth, and you deserve to have every advantage you can get on your way to the perfect bridal body.

You might be surprised, but when it comes to burning fat and sculpting an impressive physique, I've found what you eat day in and day out has more of an impact than exercise alone. I'd say that nutrition makes up about 70-75% of any fat loss plan.

Now, I'm not saying forget about exercise, what I'm saying is that you need BOTH to get optimal results. In an article titled "Metabolism Makeover" by Dr. Len Kravitz, those who dieted *only* and did not exercise actually had a decrease in their metabolism. Those who dieted *and* exercised were able to continue losing weight while preventing a metabolism drop, and keep calories burning even while eating fewer calories. Keep that in mind when we get to the next chapter on workouts.

What I am saying is that if you want to lose weight, instead of just cutting back on calories, you really need to focus on the quality of those calories. When you do this, you will find that you'll feel fuller, and it's a way of eating you can stick with, all while losing weight and burning fat!

Diets suck. This is NOT a DIET!

Before I explain what you'll be eating with the meal plans, I want to first explain why this method is not like most other "diets".

Dieting SUCKS.

You are starving yourself and depriving your body of calories and nutrients. It is a period of voluntary starvation when you think about it. Companies create these programs that limit what you can eat, hoping that you'll just say "OK, this sounds awesome, totally pumped to get anorexic!"

On top of these diets "sucking", the numbers show that 90% of people who start a diet will not stick it out in a year. If you've dieted before, you probably know that it's hard to stick to one. The problem I see is that if something isn't working for 90% of people, then there is something wrong with the diet, not the majority of people.

Think about it. If 90% of iPhones stopped working after a month, no one would sit at home and sulk thinking, "Wow, I don't know what I did wrong. I must be really awful, because my phone stopped working". Yet, what's interesting is, most people blame themselves when they are not able to make a diet "work". That's not fair to you, and it's not fair to your body. It's complete BS and you need to get out of that mindset now. The main issue is that these diets are just not sustainable. If you can't sustain a diet, I don't care how well "designed" or "researched" it is, it will not work for you.

The meal plan in this book is not so much a diet as it is a delicious way of eating healthier. At the same time, it will help you to lean out and shape a sexy new you.

Slimming superfoods: Eat more, burn more

When you fill your meals with superfoods, you create a healthier you from the inside out, while shedding fat and getting leaner. They are the foods that you should be eating at every meal, replacing junk and processed, with natural and nutritious.

Superfoods got its name, because they contain antioxidants, minerals, vitamins, fiber, protein, and healthy fats, all while maintaining a relatively low calorie count. So you are able to fill up and get all these natural benefits the way nature intended it. They are dense in nutrients, but not calories. These are the foods that you need to build a sustainable daily diet you can stick to. (And like we've already discovered, fat loss is all about being able to stick to a new diet.)

Our favorite superfoods

Let's just check out some of the superfoods that make up the meal plans and why they are so awesome for you:

Vegetables: These will fill you up with very little calories and are ESSENTIAL to weight loss. For example, according to www. whfoods.com, 1 cup of raw broccoli has over 135% of your Vitamin C, tons of Vitamin K, Folate, and lots of antioxidants, which have been shown to prevent cancer, all for under 30 calories!

Nuts & Seeds: Excellent sources of fiber, protein, and healthy fats. Some are even high in omega 3s (i.e. walnuts, flax, chia, and hemp seeds), which can prevent heart disease and keep your blood sugar levels in check. Pumpkin seeds are also full of protein and mineral selenium (brazil nuts too) that promote thyroid health. (That's critical if you want a healthy metabolism.)

Lean Meats and Fish: Wild fish, lean chicken, and grass fed beef are excellent protein sources, which help to promote muscle repair for a toned body. Studies like the 2010 article, "A review of fatty acid profiles and antioxidant content in grass-fed and grain-fed beef", actually show that grass fed beef is an excellent source of heart healthy omega 3 fatty acids, and like fish, can actually lower your cholesterol levels!

Yogurt: A great source of very high quality protein, yogurt has around 50% of your daily iodine needs. Why is this important? Iodine is necessary for thyroid health, and a healthy thyroid means a healthy metabolism (and a healthy metabolism means a skinnier you).

Berries: Low in calories, berries of all kinds are full of antioxidants that can prevent certain cancers. They are loaded with fiber to keep you full, and have a low glycemic index, so your blood sugar levels don't spike, causing cravings. (They seem to be berry good for you! I'm sorry I couldn't help myself on that one.)

Getting Lean with the Meal Plans:

Using the meal plans to shed fat, and reveal sleek and sexy body for your wedding!

Here I'll go over what makes up the meal plans and answer some questions you might have about them.

1) How many meals should I eat per day?

Is eating 6 smaller meals really better for fat loss than 3 larger meals spread out? Maybe not. In a position stand in the *International Society of Sports Nutrition*, researchers found, "Increased meal frequency does not appear to significantly enhance diet induced thermogenesis, total energy expenditure, or resting metabolic rate". So eating more frequently DOES NOT appear to "boost" the metabolism like we've been told for years.

Plus, who has time to prepare and eat 6 times a day?

In the meal plan, we get back to the basics and keep it simple with 3 meals, plus an optional snack if needed between lunch and dinner. (OR when you have the biggest gap in between meals.)

- **BREAKFAST:** Where you want to consume most of your carbs. Smoothies and Greek yogurts with fruit, or granola are great meal ideas. When in doubt, you can't go wrong with a yogurt, some nuts, and berries.

- **LUNCH:** Again, getting protein, fats, and vegetables in the lunch meal. Salads are super convenient for lunch, and you'll see that we've included a variety to choose from.

- **SNACK:** This is optional and designed to keep you satisfied if you need it. If you don't get hungry in-between lunch and dinner, then skip it!

- **DINNER:** Think more protein and less carbs. You also
  want to eat before 8pm. The later at night you eat, studies
  show the more indiscriminate you become in eating.
  Which means, you will eat whatever is in front of you.
  Don't get sucked into this trap. Eat earlier in the day
  so that you don't come home famished and start eating
  everything in sight.

2) The 3 things you should eat at EVERY meal to lose weight

If you want to shed fat and flatten your stomach, then there are
certain things you'll want to eat at every meal:

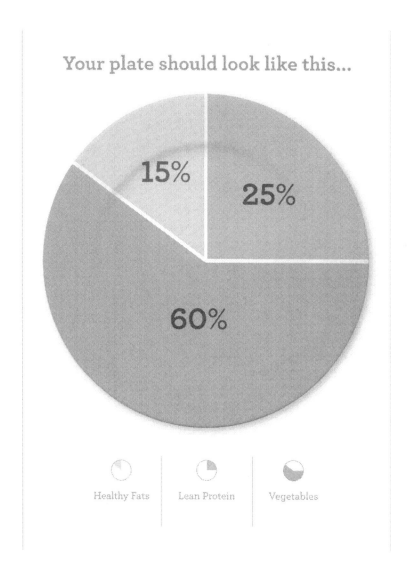

Your plate should look like this...

1. **Lean Protein:** Grilled chicken breast, eggs, fish, low fat Greek yogurt, seeds & nuts, lean ground beef, and lean ground lamb.

WHY: Lean protein helps keep you full and supports lean tissue, which will keep your metabolism burning. Don't believe me?

In a 2012 review that looked at over 24 studies, researchers at the University of South Australia compared results of standard protein and high protein diets with the total calories remaining the same. They found those eating higher protein diets lost more weight, and **specifically more fat**, while resulting in greater satiety for the majority of the studies.

This means that a higher protein diet led to more weight loss (with more of that weight loss being from fat), while keeping individuals feeling fuller for longer when compared to those who ate lower levels of protein, but the same amount of calories.

2. **Vegetables (fruit):** Broccoli, kale, squash, tomatoes, spinach, arugula, mixed greens, green beans, bell peppers, onions, etc.

WHY: Vegetables provide the bulk, the fiber, and so many of the vitamins and minerals that our body not only needs, but craves.

Quick story, one of my clients had a 2 week conference to attend, and she didn't really have much time for exercise. I was a little concerned about her; however, when she got back to the gym, she was noticeably leaner. I asked her what she had done.

She said, "Well I didn't have much time for exercise, and the food there was awful, so I just loaded up on vegetables for most of my meals." Man, did it work! She had dropped a few pounds, most of it being fat! For me, this just reinforced the importance of vegetables for fat loss.

What about fruits? Fruits do have more sugars; therefore, a higher caloric content, so we keep those limited to breakfast for the most part. Keep it to 1 serving/day of fruit at most for fat loss.

3. **Healthy Fats:** Olive oil, nuts and seeds, avocado, and cold water fish.

WHY: If you want to shed fat, then you need to be eating healthy fats. Trust me; the results are amazing! Dietary fat is CRITICAL for satiety, brain function, immune system health, and weight loss. By increasing your healthy fat intake, you receive more omega 3s so you can stay leaner, healthier, and decrease inflammation.

(Side note: Scientists estimate that about 90% of Americans DON'T eat enough Omega 3 fatty acids in their diet. Top sources include: fish, flaxseeds, walnuts, and grass fed beef.

While the meals in the meal plans have all the protein, healthy fats, and veggies built in, keep these guidelines in mind when you have to go out to eat, or are making your own recipes.

3) Carb cycling: You can still eat carbs!

While many diets are "low carb", you won't have to give up carbs on this plan. The meal plans cycle through lower and higher carb days in order to fuel your fat shedding workouts and keep your metabolic fire burning strong.

Low Carb vs. Low Fat:

In a 2004 study, "A Low-Carbohydrate, Ketogenic Diet versus a Low-Fat Diet To Treat Obesity and Hyperlipidemia: A Randomized, Controlled Trial", Dr. Yancy found that of the 120 individuals studied, **those who followed the low carb diet lost 20.7 lbs, while those who followed a low fat diet lost only 10.6 lbs.** by then end of the 24 week study even though **they ate the same amount of calories.**

On top of the increased fat loss, the low carb group had a better retention rate, meaning they found it easier to stick to the diet, and also had improved blood triglyceride levels and healthier cholesterol levels compared to the low fat group!

Carb cycling: How to do it

Ok, so lower carb diets are great, but we also need some higher carb days in there to fuel the workouts and keep your metabolism guessing, which is why you'll cycle between lower and higher carb days.

You'll just follow the meal plans and see which days are labeled lower or higher carb days. For those days, the meals are designed to conform to lower or higher carb days. Follow them and you'll be all set!

You will receive the fat burning results of a low carb diet, which can be sustained for longer than just a few weeks, and bam! That's where you get the real results.

Weekly Carb Cycling Example:

Carb Cycle

Monday	Tuesday	Wednesday	Thursday	Friday	Saturday	Sunday
Higher Carb	Lower Carb	Higher Carb	Lower Carb	Higher Carb	Cheat Day!	Lower Carb

What if I want to eat a different meal from the meal plan?

If you decide to make your own meals or swap meals from different days, make sure that they fall under the carb level for that day. Say it's Monday and you want to switch out the lunch for a different lunch from throughout the week. As Monday is a Higher Carb day, you'll want to choose a lunch from another Higher Carb day, Wednesday or Friday as an example.

Higher Carb Foods: Fruit, granola, rice, bread, quinoa, or any starchy vegetable like potato or sweet potato.

Lower Carb Foods: Most Non starchy vegetables, (spinach, broccoli, onions, tomatoes etc.) any lean proteins, nuts or seeds, cheese, olive oil.

Smash through weight loss plateaus!

As we get closer to the end of the 12 weeks, the meal plans will actually shift so that there are more Lower Carb days each week, and fewer Higher Carb days, in order to maximize the fat loss and keep from hitting any fat loss plateaus.

That being said, if you need to lose more weight, and want faster results, following the meal plan layout from weeks 9-12 for the entire 12 weeks will help you shed the pounds faster… if you are up to the challenge.

4) No calorie counting: Why counting calories is a waste of time

I'm not a big fan of counting calories for most people. Many who start a calorie counting program will give up, because it's just too much to keep up with, and I don't blame them. It's just not sustainable for most people, and if something is not sustainable, then they'll probably quit after a week.

Secondly, the whole system of calories and how they were calculated is based off an old and antiquated system that doesn't actually take into account the digestibility of certain foods and their calories, especially based on how they are prepared. So while a certain food may contain say 100 calories, the body is only able to digest 70 or 80 of those calories. Different foods have different caloric levels once ingested and digested, so to compare say, 100 calories of a cookie to 100 calories of grass fed ground beef, is really like comparing apples to oranges. (No pun intended...actually it was.)

Thirdly, many of the times **the amount of calories you see listed on a food label is NOT the actual amount of calories in the food!** In the study, "The Accuracy of Stated Energy Contents of Reduced-Energy, Commercially Prepared Foods" in the *Journal of the American Dietetics Association,* researchers found that prepared foods didn't have the same amount of calories as the nutrition labels had listed on the foods.

When comparing the actual calories vs. the calories listed on the food, the researchers found actual calories to be off by 8-18%, which added up to enough calories to gain 10-20 lb. in one year.

There are other estimates that the labeling on foods can over or underestimate the actual amount of calories by 25%.

That is just way too much error to get any accurate readings, so what's the point of counting fake numbers that may not even have any validity in the first place? Instead of focusing so much on every single calorie, you should focus on getting super high quality natural foods, and loading up on vegetables and lean proteins.

So how much SHOULD you eat?

You might be asking, "If I don't count calories, how do I know how much to eat!?" I'm going to give you a simple yet revolutionary answer, and it's a solution that you'll be able to use forever, even after the wedding if you feel like it!

Eat enough until you feel satisfied

When you have the combination of the lean protein, the healthy fats, and the vegetables, you can't help but feel full, and your body will tell you how much you need. If you are ever hungry after a meal, you can always load up on extra vegetables. (A whole 2 cups of broccoli has around 50 calories, and I dare you to eat 2 cups and still feel hungry.)

(NOTE: If your plate if full of vegetables and you are eating slower, then your stomach will be feeling full before you have the chance to fill it with a huge amount of calories. This is how this system works.)

If you are drinking enough water, this will also help to keep you feeling full throughout the day, especially if you are drinking water before meals. Which brings us to hydration.

When in doubt, add more vegetables. No one ever got fat eating broccoli!

5) Hydration: Drinking yourself slimmer!

- **WATER:**

Listen, if you want to lose weight (and keep burning fat) you need to stay hydrated. The female body is made up of around 60-65% water. Everything you do requires water, including metabolism and digestion. If you neglect your water intake, do you really think your body is going to be an efficient fat burning machine you want it to be?

(This is also the reason it is so easy to drop "weight" quickly when you dehydrate yourself. You may weigh less on a scale, but you won't look or feel any better when you lose water weight using "lose weight fast" diets.)

Make water your best friend, and you'll start to see results. **One of the main habits of those who have transformed their physiques and maintained their new bodies is the habit of drinking water regularly, carrying around water with them throughout the day.** Another related habit they also share is not drinking their calories. This means avoiding juices, sodas, and any other type of calorie containing drink.

If you want to be super slim, stick to the meal plans and when it comes to drinks, keep it to water, unsweetened green tea, and coffee.

How much water should you drink?

Hydration is key to losing weight and keeping it off. So the rule is to **drink half your body weight in ounces per day.**

This means that if you are 140 lbs., you would cut that in half, and end up at 70 fluid oz. for the day. 1 cup is 8 oz., so you would need almost 10 cups of water as a general rule.

- **WATER EQUATION: 1/2 x (your Weight) = The amount of fluid ounces of water you need each day.**

Note: A good way to know if you are hydrated enough is as simple as checking the color of your urine. It should be a clear color, as opposed to a darker apple juice like color.

- **Soda and Juice:**

Imagine soda and fruit juices as being like drugs. Just say no. Any drinks that contain calories should be limited. Juice is not as healthy as eating the actual fruit, as its been stripped of the fiber. Studies have also shown that solid foods will help keep you fuller when compared to liquids containing the same amount of calories. Eat your food, don't drink it.

- **Alcohol:**

Alcohol in no way leads to fat loss. It is just added calories. That being said, I'm always asked, "But what about red wine, I heard it's good for you!" Yes, it does contain antioxidants that studies have shown are helpful and healthy, and heck, who doesn't enjoy a nice glass of wine with dinner.

If you are going to drink, keep it to red wine, (white is more sugary) and keep it to 1-2 glasses TOPS. I'm giving you some leeway here, but don't go overboard with it. If you consume a whole bottle, then you're on your own. You'll be ruining your results, and probably feeling like crap in the morning.

6) Cheat meals: You don't have to give up anything!

By including some of your favorite foods each week in a scheduled "cheat meal" you'll be able to satisfy any cravings you have, while at the same time refreshing you physically and mentally. You might be thinking, "This makes no sense. Shouldn't I be eating super clean and healthy ALL the time?"

Listen, I know it sounds counterintuitive, but whether or not you plan it, you will most likely end up eating 1 or 2 meals per week that don't quite fit the meal plan.

If you are sticking to the meal plan each week, then 1 or 2 meals will NOT derail your progress, in fact my clients who regularly included a "cheat meal" or two, each week were the ones sticking with the program the longest. They had better results over time, because they were able to keep going with the plan.

How to cheat: Start off healthy, and then reward yourself

Each Saturday, you'll see that there are 2 cheat meals on the meal plan. Start off with a healthy breakfast, then eat whatever you've been craving, for lunch and dinner. You can eat any food, but not any amount. If you've been dreaming of pizza all week, have a slice or two tops, but not the whole pie. Make sense?

Now if you see that your results are coming a bit slow, you might want to limit it to 1 cheat meal per week. And your cheat meal doesn't have to be unhealthy; one of my clients loves sushi, and so that's what she treats herself to. It's really up to you. Some weeks I eat a cheat meal, some weeks I don't. See what works best for you.

7) Foods to avoid: The foods making you fat!

We've talked about what foods you want to eat to lose, but that only works if you're also cutting out the foods that are making you fat. There are certain foods that just don't belong in your diet if you hope to achieve the bridal body of your dreams.

Nowadays, we are surrounded by pre-made "foods" that are nothing more than carbohydrate rich, nutrient deficient products loaded with preservatives. **I won't even refer to them as food, seriously.**

In order to get that slim and sexy body for your wedding, you need to avoid the foods that have been holding you back. I've listed below the "foods" that you want to avoid at all costs if you want to lean out and finally lose that fat.

- **Drinks: Any Alcohol, Carbonated drinks, Soda, or Juices**

Like we said, any sodas will prevent your fat loss. Alcohol is another killer. Juice, while seemingly healthy, is very easy to consume quickly and often lacks the fiber and other nutrients that come with eating whole fruits and vegetables. Stick to water, green teas, and coffee. Milks are to be used for smoothies, but not as drink for this program.

- **Soy Products**

While soy was originally touted as a health food, recent studies are showing that certain components of soy may actually lead to certain types of breast cancer, due to its ability to act like estrogen in the body. For these reasons, I advise my bridal clients (and everyone for that matter) that it's smart to stay away from soy. I'm not saying soy will give you cancer, but why risk the possibility when there are higher quality protein sources out there?

- **Anything Packaged**

"If it's packaged, it's usually no good" is our motto at the Wedding Gym. If something is packaged, it's usually a processed food, which has been stripped of its nutrients, and loaded with sodium so it can last for months, if not years on the grocery shelves. Ditch these in favor of fresh and natural foods if you want a killer body for your wedding.

- **Anything Fake**

More and more, natural foods are being shown to be much healthier than our man made versions. Instead of fat free salad dressings, go with all natural versions that use full fat olive oil. Instead of fake butter, go with Kerrygold Irish Butter. It's made from cows that are grass fed, so it contains healthier fats.

- **Too Much Fruit?**

Ok, before you think I'm crazy, I'm not saying fruit is bad. Fruit is good, but TOO MUCH fruit can hold back fat loss. People have been told that fruit is healthy, so they eat 4-5 servings a day, when they should be eating more vegetables and keeping fruit intake to 1.5-2 servings MAX in order to shed fat. You should aim to eat the fruit around the time you work out, either before or after, as your sugar needs increase with more intense exercise.

Make sure to remove these foods from your daily diet if you really want to burn that fat. Could you have them during your cheat meal each week, sure, but if you can avoid it, do so. These things don't have a place in the body of a healthy, slim and sexy bride-to-be.

8)   The extras: ketchup and chocolate?

I always get questions about these 2 things, condiments and chocolate. "What kind of sauces or condiments can I eat?" or "What about chocolate? I've heard it's good for you!"

Ok, first I'll go over the condiments; some you can use in moderation, and some you want to avoid altogether.

Good To Go Condiments: These you can use liberally throughout the day.

- Natural Vinaigrette

- Cinnamon

- Black pepper

* Cumin

* Paprika

* Basil

* Hot Sauce (Tabasco is a good low sodium choice)

* Ginger

* Mustards

* Any Low Sodium Seasonings or Spices (Mrs. Dash is great)

* Lime or Lemon Juice (Really good on meats and salads!)

Condiments in Moderation: Use sparingly each day.

* Ketchup and BBQ Sauce (Higher Carb days) 1-2 tbsp.

* Salt, use a pinch

* Kerrygold Butter, less than 1 oz.

* Honey

* Agave

Condiments to Avoid: These should be avoided most of the time, if not all the time.

* Artificial Salad Dressings

* Any Creamy Sauces

* Soy Sauces (High Sodium)

* Fake Mayonnaise

* Margarine

- Anything fake, "Fat Free", "Sugar Free", and anything labeled "Free". These are artificial.

What about chocolate?

One small square of dark chocolate for dessert won't destroy your lean body results, and it does contain certain antioxidants and flavanols, which studies suggest can decrease your risk of heart disease and lower blood pressure. Like everything else, keep it in moderation. An entire bar each day will only set your weight loss goals back further.

Stick with a square inch piece of dark chocolate after dinner to satisfy cravings, and not ruin your hard earned physique.

Go Dark and Natural: The more chocolate is processed, the more the flavanols are destroyed, so get it as natural as you can. Keep it dark, around 70% dark chocolate is where you will gain the most benefits without too much extra sugar and fat that comes from milk chocolate.

The Meal Plans

Without further ado, here are the meal plans for the next 12 weeks. You'll see that there are lots of different meals for each day. If you like certain meals more than another, feel free to eat them on other days, just make sure that if it's a Higher Carb meal, you are eating it on a Higher Carb day.

Grocery Lists are provided in the "Extras" section at the back of the book, where you'll also find the Kitchen Makeover Manual to help you get your kitchen prepped and ready to begin your bridal body transformation.

Phase One: Week 2, 3, & 4:

MEALS	Monday High Carb	Tuesday Low Carb	Wednesday High Carb	Thursday Low Carb
Breakfast	**Pear & Avocado Smoothie** 1 ripe pear 1/2 cup berries 1/4 avocado 1 cup almond milk 1/2 cup water **Add vanilla extract or cinnamon to taste.**	**Greek Yogurt & Granola** 1 cup low-fat greek yogurt 1/2 cup granola **Add cinnamon to taste.**	**Berries & Oatmeal** 1 cup oatmeal 1 cup low fat milk 2/3 cup strawberries **Add some honey and cinnamon to taste.**	**Feta Eggs & Broccoli** 2 scrambled eggs 1 cup steamed broccoli 1 cup mangoes chopped 1 tbsp. feta cheese crumbles **Top eggs with feta, serve with broccoli and mangoes.**
Lunch	**Lime Chicken and Rice** 4 oz. grilled Chicken breast 1 cup steamed broccoli 1/2 cup brown rice 2 tbsp. olive oil 1/2 lime **Squeeze lime on chicken and rice, drizzle olive oil, salt & pepper to taste.**	**Avocado & Tomato Salad** 2 cups mixed greens 1/2 avocado sliced 1 cup cherry tomatoes 1 tbsp. vinaigrette **Mix together and salt pepper to taste.**	**Mango Greek Yogurt & Almonds** 1 cup low-fat plain Greek yogurt 1 cup mango chunks 1/4 cup or 10 almonds **Mix yogurt with mangoes and top with almonds.**	**Spinach Salad W/ Chicken** 2 cups baby spinach 4oz grilled chicken 1 tbsp. chopped red onion 1 tbsp. olive oil **Mix together and add grated parmesan and black pepper to taste.**
Snack	Apple	**Small handful of pumpkin seeds**	**Small handful of almonds**	**1-2 tbsp. Almond butter**
Dinner	**Dijon Grilled Chicken & Rice** 4oz grilled chicken breast 2 cups of spinach ½ cup sautéed onions & bell peppers 1-2 tbsp. olive oil ½ cup of brown rice Dijon mustard **Use Dijon mustard as a sauce for the chicken.**	**Greek Lamb Burger** 4oz lean ground lamb 1 tomato sliced 1 cup steamed broccoli 1 oz. feta cheese **Mix ground lamb and feta together, and cook. Then serve with tomato slices and broccoli. Drizzle olive oil over broccoli.**	**Grilled Chicken & Sweet Potato** 4 oz. grilled chicken breast 1 cup steamed broccoli 1 baked sweet potato 1-2 tablespoons of olive oil Optional: hot sauce **Drizzle olive oil and hot sauce over chicken and broccoli.**	**Hummus and Veggies** ½ cup of hummus 1 cup of steamed broccoli ½ bell pepper (fresh) 1 cup carrots **Enjoy all vegetables with hummus.**

MEALS	Friday High Carb	Saturday Cheat Day	Sunday Low Carb
Breakfast	**Mango Smoothie** 1 cup mango chunks 1 cup chopped kale 1.5 cup coconut or almond milk 1/4 cup sunflower seeds **Combine all and blend until smooth.**	**Greek Yogurt & Blueberries** 1 cup low-fat greek yogurt 1 cup blueberries 1/4 cup pumpkin seeds **Mix yogurt and berries, top with pumpkin seeds.**	Pick from any day.
Lunch	**Quinoa Salad** 1 cup quinoa 1 cup broccoli 1/2 cup sautéed onions and bell peppers 1 tbsp. olive oil **Mix all ingredients together and serve.**	**Cheat Meal: Whatever you want!**	Choose from Tues or Thurs
Snack	Lara Bar	(Optional)	Choose from Tues or Thurs
Dinner	**Grilled Lemon Fish** 4 oz. grilled wild white fish 2 cups fresh baby spinach or kale 1-2 tbsp. olive oil ½ lemon **Drizzle olive oil over spinach and rice or quinoa; squeeze lemon juice over grilled fish.**	**Cheat Meal: Whatever you want!**	Choose from Tues or Thurs

Phase Two: Weeks 5-8:

MEALS	Monday Moderate Carb	Tuesday Low Carb	Wed High Carb	Thursday Low Carb
Breakfast	**Strawberry Granola** 1 cup low-fat milk ½ cup granola 1 cup strawberries **Top granola with strawberries, and milk.**	**Blueberry Protein Smoothie** 1 cup blueberries 1 scoop vanilla protein 1.5 cup almond or coconut milk 1 tbsp. of almond butter **Blend all together.**	**Cheesy Eggs & Blueberries** 2 scrambled eggs (1 yolk removed) 1 cup steamed broccoli 1 oz. of cheese ½ cup of blueberries (fresh) (Use hot sauce instead of ketchup) Let cheese melt on top of eggs before serving.	**Peach Oatmeal** 1 cup oatmeal 1 cup low fat milk 2/3 cup berries, (strawberries or blueberries) **Cook oatmeal with milk and add berries on top, drizzle some honey and add a dash of cinnamon.**
Lunch	**Greek Yogurt & Orange** 1 cup low-fat greek yogurt 1 navel orange 1/4 cup raw cashews **Enjoy.**	**SuperFood Salad** 2 cups of mixed greens 2 cups mixed vegetables ¼ cup sunflower seeds 2 tbsp. olive oil 1 tbsp. feta or goat cheese **Mix all together, use black pepper to taste.**	**Greek Quinoa Salad** ½ cup cooked quinoa 2 cups baby spinach fresh 1 cup broccoli, steamed 1 plum tomato chopped 1 oz. feta cheese 1 tbsp. olive oil **Mix all together and serve on spinach, black pepper to taste.**	**Chicken Avocado Salad** -3-4 oz. grilled chicken breast -½ avocado sliced thin -2 cups baby spinach, fresh -1 cup cherry tomatoes, sliced -1 tbsp. olive oil (hot sauce optional) **Mix all together and add dash of black pepper.**
Snack	10 raw almonds	1/2 cup sunflower seeds	1 apple or pear	1/4 cup of pumpkin seeds
Dinner	**Grilled Chicken Parm** 4 oz. grilled chicken breast 1 tomato, sliced 1 cups of spinach with 1 cup broccoli, steamed 1 oz. mozzarella, sliced thin 1 tbsp. olive oil **Cut tomato into halves and cook in olive oil, top chicken with tomatoes and mozzarella slices. Drizzle olive oil on spinach. Add pepper to taste.**	**Chipotle Burger*** 4 oz. grass fed beef 2 cups arugula ½ tomato sliced ½ chipotle pepper, chopped 1 tbsp. adobo sauce from can 1-2 tbsp. olive oil **Mix chopped chipotle pepper with beef to make burger patty and cook. Top with tomato slices and adobo sauce from chipotle can. Drizzle olive oil and pepper over arugula. *Spicy**	**Hummus & Stir-fry** ½ bell pepper, sliced ¼ cup chopped onion ½ cup chopped zucchini 1 tbsp. olive oil ¼ cup hummus 1 medium sized pita bread **Cook all veggies together in a frying pan with olive oil. Then serve with hummus & pita bread.**	**Grilled Lime Fish** 4 oz. grilled wild white fish ½ cup rice or quinoa 1 cup fresh baby spinach or kale 2 tbsp. olive oil ½ lemon **Drizzle olive oil over spinach and rice or quinoa; squeeze lime juice over grilled fish.**

MEALS	Friday High Carb	Saturday Cheat Day	Sunday Low Carb
Breakfast	**Orange Creamsicle Smoothie** 1 cup vanilla low fat Greek yogurt 1 orange 1.5 cups water 2 tbsp. chia seeds 1/2 tsp. Vanilla extract **Blend until all smooth.**	**Pear & Avocado Smoothie** 1 ripe pear 1/2 cup berries 1/4 avocado 1 cup almond milk 1/2 cup water **Add vanilla extract or cinnamon to taste.**	Choose from any days this week
Lunch	**Greek Quinoa Salad** ½ cup cooked quinoa 2 cups baby spinach fresh 1 cup broccoli, steamed 1 plum tomato chopped 1 oz. feta cheese 1 tbsp. olive oil **Mix all together and serve on spinach. Black pepper to taste**	**Cheat Meal: Whatever you want!**	Choose from Tues or Thurs
Snack	1 tbsp. almond butter	(Optional)	Choose from Tues or Thurs
Dinner	**Lemon Mustard Chicken** 4 oz. grilled chicken breast 2 cups mixed greens 1 cup broccoli 1/4 avocado, sliced 1 tbsp. Dijon mustard 1 tbsp. lemon juice **Mix mustard, lemon juice and olive oil together and coat chicken breast, then cook chicken. Serve sliced avocado and drizzle with lemon juice with chicken and broccoli on spinach.**	**Cheat Meal: Whatever you want!**	Choose from Tues or Thurs

Phase Three: Weeks 9-12:

MEALS	Monday Moderate Carb	Tuesday Low Carb	Wednesday Higher Carb	Thursday Low Carb
Breakfast	**Blueberry-Almond Smoothie** 1 cup blueberries 1 cup coconut milk 1 cup water 1 tbsp. of almond butter 1 tbsp. chia seeds 1 tsp. honey Dash of cinnamon **Blend all together until smooth.**	**Raspberry Greek Yogurt** 1 cup low-fat greek yogurt ¼ cup granola 1 cup of raspberries **Mix berries into yogurt and top granola and a dash of cinnamon**	**Eggs & Fruit** 2 scrambled eggs ½ cup of pinto beans ½ cup berries **Serve beans with eggs, use hot sauce if you'd like.**	**Blueberry Granola** 1 cup coconut milk beverage ½ cup granola 1 cup blueberries **Top granola with strawberries, and milk. Dash of cinnamon on top.**
Lunch	**Greek Yogurt** 1 cup low-fat Greek yogurt 1 pear ¼ cup cashews (1 handful) **Add a dash of cinnamon to yogurt.**	**Arugula Pepper Steak Salad** 4 oz. skirt or flank steak 2 cups mixed arugula and spinach 1 oz. crumbled goat or feta cheese 1 tbsp. olive oil 1 tbsp. lemon juice Dash black pepper **Cook steak and cut into thin strips. Combine arugula, walnuts, and then top with steak. Mix olive oil, lemon juice and cracked black pepper and drizzle on top.**	**Avocado-Chicken Salad** 2 cups baby spinach 4oz grilled chicken breast, sliced ¼ avocado, sliced thin ½ cup broccoli, steamed 1 tbsp. of olive oil Optional: hot sauce & black pepper **Mix all together and then top with grated hot sauce and pepper.**	**Salad w/ Grilled Chicken** 2 cups mixed greens 4 oz. grilled chicken, chopped 1 cup cherry tomatoes 1 tbsp. chopped red onions 2 tbsp. olive oil ½ tbsp. grated parmesan **Mix all together, then top with grated parmesan and black pepper.**
Snack	1/4 cup cashews	1/4 cup raw walnuts	Small handful of pumpkin seeds	1/4 cup or small handful of sunflower seeds
Dinner	**Grilled Chicken & Squash** 4 oz. grilled chicken 1 cup roasted butternut squash 1 cup kale, fresh 2 tbsp. olive oil **Drizzle olive oil over kale and squash. Salt and pepper to taste. (Very easy on the salt.)**	**Hummus and Veggies** ½ cup of hummus 2 cups mixed greens 1 cup of steamed broccoli **Serve all veggies with hummus.**	**BBQ Grilled Chicken** 4 oz. grilled chicken breast 2 cups mixed veggies, frozen ½ baked sweet potato 1 tablespoon of olive oil Optional: hot sauce **Drizzle olive oil and hot sauce over chicken.**	**Lean Lamb & Veggies** 4oz lean ground lamb ½ bell pepper sliced ¼ cup red onion chopped 2 cups steamed broccoli Dash of black pepper **Cook peppers and onions in pan with lamb, until the lamb is cooked through. Steam broccoli and serve with meat and veggies. Add Tabasco for a spicy finish once served.**

MEALS	Friday Low Carb	Saturday Cheat Day	Sunday Low Carb
Breakfast	**Pear & Avocado Smoothie** 1 pear sliced up ¼ cup berries ¼ avocado 1 cup milk (almond, coconut, low fat) 1 tsp. honey Dash of cinnamon. **Blend until smooth.** **Optional: Add dash of vanilla extract.**	**Mango-Kale Smoothie** 1 cup chopped kale 1 cup mango chunks 1 cup coconut milk beverage 1 cup water ¼ cup sunflower seeds Dash of cinnamon **Blend until fully smooth.**	**Choose from any days this week**
Lunch	**Kale & Walnut Salad** 2 cups fresh kale, chopped ¼ cup chopped walnuts 1 cup cherry tomatoes 1 cup broccoli, steamed 1-2 tbsp. of olive oil Optional: 1 tbsp. feta crumbles **Mix all together and then top with feta.**	**SuperFoods Salad** 2 cups spinach 1 carrot, chopped ¼ cup pumpkin seeds ¼ cup red onion chopped 2 tbsp. olive oil 1 tbsp. lemon juice black pepper **Combine greens and vegetables. Mix olive oil, lemon juice and pepper and drizzle on top.**	**Choose from Tues or Thurs**
Snack	1 tbsp. almond butter	(Optional)	**Choose from Tues or Thurs**
Dinner	**Spicy Lime-Avocado Chicken** 4 oz. grilled chicken breast 1/2 avocado, sliced 1 cup broccoli or mixed vegetables 1 lime, halved **Squeeze lime juice and hot sauce over grilled chicken and sliced avocado.**	**Cheat Meal: Whatever you want!**	**Choose from Tues or Thurs**

Slimming Meals Summary

- **3 Meals a day:** Eat 3 meals per day with an optional snack if you are hungry. Follow the plan each day.

- **Eat superfoods from grocery list:** Stick to the foods designed to shed the fat from your body and build a lean sculpted you. Remember, lean protein, LOTS of vegetables, and healthy fats in each meal.

- **Cheat meals:** 2x/week in the first 2 months (Phase 1 & 2), and 1x week for the last 4 weeks (Phase 3). This is your time to truly enjoy your favorite foods, but don't go overboard with portions, stay in check.

- **Protein at EVERY meal:** Higher protein intake helps burn fat. Seeds, Greek yogurt, chicken, and fish are great examples of high protein foods. Eat it if you want to lose weight.

- **Carbs:** Each day is either a Lower or Higher Carb day, and the meals reflect that.

- **Hydration:** Stay hydrated with water, teas, and coffee. Aim for ½ your bodyweight in ounces. Example: A 140 lb woman would need 70 ounces. Avoid sodas, juices, and carbonated drinks, as these will make weight loss VERY difficult.

- **Avoid the foods that will destroy your bridal body:** By avoiding processed, packaged foods, soy, too much fruit, and artificial "foods" you will be able to see your body change in a good way!

- **"Kitchen Makeover" get rid of what's not helpful, replace with winning foods:**

There's a rule, "If it's there, you will eventually eat it". Don't tempt yourself, get rid of foods that are not on the plan, AND get the foods that are on the plan. You can't eat healthy if you don't have healthy foods available!

- **Shopping 1x a week, prepping 1-2x a week:** Shopping is key to having the foods you need to create a sexy new you. Prepping the meals will make it so much easier to eat right while planning a wedding.

And number 10…

EAT ONLY WHEN YOU ARE HUNGRY, DO NOT EAT WHEN YOU ARE NOT HUNGRY.'

Why all caps? Because this is one of the most important parts of this program to lead you to a lifetime of weight loss success.

Chapter Three

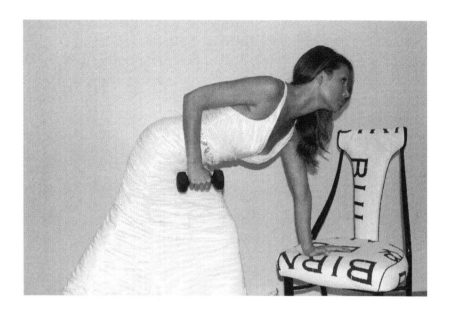

STEP 3: Sculpt & TONE

The tale of the belly pouch mystery

I had a client come to me and in our initial consult she told me, "I've been trying to get rid of this pouch here for the longest time", as she grabbed the jiggle on her belly. She was really frustrated and told me that she knew what to do, she was eating "right", she was working out all the time, but could NOT get rid of that stomach fat, which is why she called me up. With just a few questions I was pretty sure I knew what was happening.

When I asked her what she did for exercise she replied, "running". I then asked her, "What else?" She replied simply, "Well, that's about it, but I run like 4 times a week!"

BINGO. Once we introduced some resistance training and tweaked her diet, she got leaner, her body fat decreased, and that fat stomach pouch started to flatten right out. Simple as that, yet what I find is that most women still stick only to cardio and avoid resistance training like the plague when they hit the gym, and they couldn't be making a bigger mistake.

You've been lied to?

Quite simply, you haven't been told the truth about what works for fat loss. When you walk into any gym, you'll see that most women are on the cardio machines, and the guys are all lifting weights. While the women are busting out their 45-60 minutes or longer of cardio, they are missing out on some of the best exercises to sculpt and tone their bodies. Many of these women still struggle to drop the pounds, and wonder why they can't lose weight even though they are spending so much time in the gym week in and week out.

What if I told you that you that by adding in resistance work you could be burning more calories more of the time and carving out a slim and sexy body all in less than 30 minutes?

A better bridal body in less than 30 minutes

The truth is, if you want to truly change your physique, look more toned, and leaner, while shedding those pounds, then you need to incorporate resistance training into your workouts.

Doing cardio alone will NOT shape your body. Cardio will help to melt some fat covering your musculature, but it's the squats, lunges, kettlebell swings, and thrusters that will leave you with a sexy butt, thighs, arms, and stomach that you can't wait to show off. With the techniques that used in the workouts in this book, I'll show you how to shape & sculpt, while absolutely crushing calories in 30 minutes or less each day. There's no need to spend hours upon hours in the gym each week.

Realistically, even if you are working out 5 days in a week, with my workouts, you'll be spending about 3 hours MAX each week exercising, possibly less. And as a busy bride, I know you need to have the most efficient workouts possible, even if you love working out, I'm sure you have a million other things to be doing.

How resistance sculpts

This will be a quick science lesson. I'll try and make it fast, promise.

Ok, so in order to lose weight, you need to burn more calories than you are consuming. The total amount of calories you burn each day (Total Energy Expenditure or TEE) is a result of 3 factors - the digestion of food, physical activity, and your RMR (resting metabolic rate).

Here's a chart giving you a better idea of what makes up all the calories that you burn in a given day:

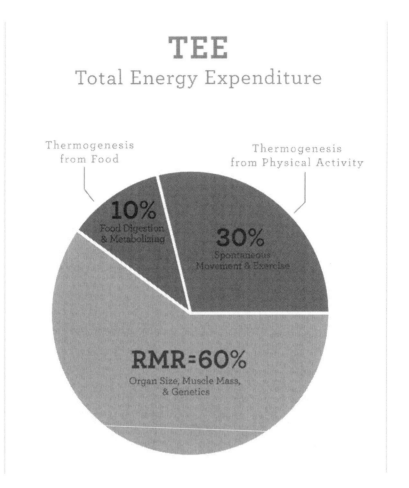

If we want the biggest impact on the amount of calories we want to burn, we quickly see that if we can affect the RMR, we will get much better results, as RMR accounts for 60% of the total amount of calories burned in 24 hours.

Attacking the RMR to supercharge fat loss

What the heck is RMR and how can we use it to boost our metabolisms?

Imagine if you just lay down in bed and didn't move for 24 hours. You would burn about 1200-1400 calories just to support activities like breathing, keeping organs running, and body temperature stable. This is the resting metabolic rate or RMR. Your RMR is determined by genetics, hormones, as well as the amount of organs like our brain, kidneys, and lean tissue like bones and muscles. Surprisingly, it takes a lot of calories just to keep you alive and not wasting away, and while we can't change the size of our brain or kidneys, we can change the amount of lean tissue we have. This is where resistance training comes in to help boost your metabolism.

Turbo charging fat loss: Resistance training

When you jump on the treadmill or elliptical, or perform any other type of cardio for that matter, you burn calories while you are exercising, but once you stop, you stop burning those calories. The calorie burning is restricted to the time you are actually exercising. With resistance training, (i.e. lifting weights and performing body weight exercises) you typically burn fewer calories during the actual exercise, but unlike regular cardio, you continue to burn calories for many hours after your workout has ended. Following resistance training, your metabolic rate is increased for hours after finishing the workout, so even when you step out of the gym you are still burning more calories compared to if you just did cardio alone. (Interestingly enough, doing higher intensity cardio intervals also leads to this increased afterburn of calories.)

On top of the more sustained calorie burning effects of resistance training, you also add some lean tissue. The more lean tissue you have, the higher your resting metabolic rate (RMR) will be. The higher your RMR, the more calories you'll be burning all day, every day. On top of an increased metabolism, you will also be shaping your body in a way that cardio can't. Cardio alone does not lead to more toned looking muscles, or a better shaped butt, this is where resistance is key.

NO you won't get huge

You won't get big unless you are taking steroids. Don't take steroids, and you'll be OK.

Women have 15-20X lower testosterone levels than men, and it's this hormone that is primarily responsible for muscle growth. So unless you are juicing (with steroids, not a juice cleanse), it will be VERY difficult for you to get huge.

Even men still need to take steroids if they want to get bodybuilder huge. So if they do have the hormone levels to support muscle growth, spend all day lifting, and still have struggles getting huge, what makes you think you will?

So NO, Lifting will NOT make you bigger......only sexier!

ALL of the workout sessions with my private bridal clients are resistance based, and the workouts found in this book are all based on workouts that I use with my clients. It works and that's why I use it.

My 4 wedding workout staples:

Here I'll explain my 4 secrets to sculpting a sexy body. These are the exact techniques I use with my clients ... Let's check 'em out.

1)   **Resistance Training**

2)   **Circuit Training**

3)   **Full Body Moves**

4)   **Posture Training**

1) Resistance training:

It's no secret that resistance training is super effective for sculpting a bridal body. I use resistance with ALL of my clients. Whether it's a medicine ball, dumbbell, or your own body weight, you'll be using resistance to sculpt your way to a sexier body. One of my favorite resistance exercise is kettlebell swings, and for good reason. I use them with all my clients, especially when we are pressed for time. They deliver great full body workouts that really burn the calories and challenge the whole body, a perfect fusion of resistance and cardio all in one exercise! In addition to the fat burning effects you get working with kettlebells, you'll also be working all the muscles that help to reverse the postural damage we do by sitting all day long. **It's THE bridal exercise.**

In fact, a recent study showed that those doing kettlebell exercises burned calories at a rate much higher than high intensity cardio, **burning 400 calories in a 20 minute session!** And while they were using an advanced move (the kettlebell snatch) you can see that there is still a lot of potential for serious fat burning when you use the kettlebell.

Here's a chart that compares kettlebell workouts vs. other popular cardio workouts:

Calories Burned in 60 min. with Various Exercises (140lb Woman)

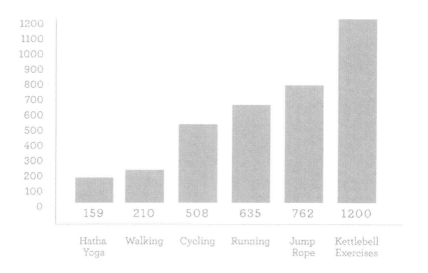

159	210	508	635	762	1200
Hatha Yoga	Walking	Cycling	Running	Jump Rope	Kettlebell Exercises

Finish a circuit of KB swings, and you'll know that you are getting a serious workout, burning calories with every swing! Plain and simple … if you want to seriously sculpt out a new body, then you want to use kettlebells.

2) Circuit training:

Without getting fancy, circuit training is nothing more than performing several exercises back to back in a workout. Again, it's what the top trainers use to get great results in half the time. If you want to shed more fat and tone up quicker, then you'll be smart to do the same. Instead of doing one exercise, resting, and then performing it again and then resting again (you can see how time consuming this could be), you would perform an exercise, like a squat, and then move right into another exercise, like a push up. It gets your heart rate up like you're doing cardio, sculpts your muscles, and reduces workout time considerably.

Studies show that those exercising using a circuit based program **lose more body fat** than those working out in a traditional format, and it's no surprise! That's why I've made the workouts entirely circuit based. This keeps you slimming down for the gown in the shortest amount of time possible!

3) Full body moves:

The third component of the workouts is usage of full body movements. This means that all of the workouts use exercises that tap into multiple muscles of the body to burn the maximal amount of calories, creating a sculpting and toning environment on your body from head to toe. Besides burning more calories, full body exercises work the whole body in less time, shortening your workouts and making them even more efficient.

4) Posture: The key to a beautiful bridal body.

Let's face it, you'll have hundreds, if not thousands, of pictures taken at your wedding, and I'm just guessing, but I think you'll want to look the best you can in every one. This is why we include postural work with one of the most effective exercises for "Princess Perfect" posture.

When a study compared women with good and bad postures, those who had better postures appeared taller, slimmer, younger, and more attractive than those with bad postures. (Even though those women with bad postures were the same height, and actually **weighed less** than those women with the good posture!)

To create a complete and well-balanced workout, the band hold exercise is included in every warm-up of the workouts. If you have issues with posture, then I would recommend doing these every day, not just on the workout days. You really can't overdo it with the postural band holds, and the more you do, the better!

The Workouts:

How to use the workouts

You'll see that there are 3 days of resistance workouts each week, and we've designed them to be on Monday, Wednesday, and Friday. For greater fat loss, we recommend cardio days in between, and you'll see we've included them on Tuesdays and Thursdays. This will give your body a day of recovery in-between each resistance workout, while also burning some extra calories. You don't want to do the resistance workouts 2 days in a row. Let your body rest and recover, as this is when your body can repair and get the most out of each workout. For the cardio days, keep it to a simple workout of 30 minutes, whether it's running, biking, rowing, swimming, jumping rope, etc. We've included an interval workout you can perform on these days in the "extras" page www.weddinggym.com/bookextras.

Weekly work out schedule

Monday	Tuesday	Wednesday	Thursday	Friday	Saturday	Sunday
Day 1: Resistance Workout	Day 2: Cardio 30 Min	Day 3: Core & Conditioning	Day 4: Cardio 30 Min	Day 5: Resistance Workout	Day 6: Rest optional Cardio 30 min	Day 7: Rest

Starting off: Test Days

The very first workout of the program will be the initial Test Day outlined in the Assessments Section of this book. From week 2 and on, you will follow the calendar above, again, you can get access to a full workout calendar on www.weddinggym.com/bookextras.

Resistance training days

- **Day 1**, or Monday, you'll see that the kettlebell swings are always there, and that's because they are so effective and efficient. Don't worry if at first you don't get the hang of them, as the weeks progress you'll do more and more of them, becoming better and better as you go.

- **Day 3, or** Wednesday, is the Core and Conditioning Day where the workouts focus on full body conditioning to burn fat and target the core while toning from head to toe.

- **Day 5, or** Friday, of each week will incorporate full body resistance and core work. Like we mentioned before, on Weeks 4, 8, and 12, Day 5 (Friday) will be the Test Day, which replaces the Friday workout that week. (Don't worry about missing the workout, if you are pushing yourself as hard as you should be on the testing day, you'll be getting more than enough of a workout that day.)

- For video on how to do the swings, and full workout calendar go to www.weddinggym.com/bookextras

Cardio Days: Tuesdays, Thursdays, & Optional Saturday

- **Type:** Running, rowing, and jumping rope burn crazy calories, low impact options include biking, rowing, or elliptical. So if you have any nagging injuries, those might be better options. Try switching it up from week to week to avoid boredom and keep your results from plateauing.

- **Intensity:** If you are a beginner to exercise, start off at an easier pace and work your way up each week, pushing harder and faster as you become more comfortable. If you are more experienced, you can try doing interval work for the cardio. An example would be doing 1 minute at a fast pace, and then taking 1-2 minutes at an easy pace to recover before starting back up with the high intensity pace for the 1 minute and so-on. Repeat this process for the 30 minutes.

- **Length:** 30 minutes tops for interval work, 30-45 minutes if you are going at a moderate pace (you are sweating and breathing so that you would not be able to hold a conversation).

- **Saturday:** If you are looking to burn even more calories and melt more fat, try adding an extra cardio day on Saturday.

(NOTE: If you are not trying to lose more weight, then do not do any extra cardio on Saturday.)

Reading and understanding the workouts

You'll have changing workouts as you move from one month to the next in the plan, which prevents your body from getting used to certain moves. Below I've listed some terms that you'll find in the workouts. If you are new to exercise, then knowing what these terms mean will help you understand how the workouts will work.

- **Warm-up:** Each workout starts with the Warm-Up, which you will perform first before moving on to the main workout circuits.

and more toned you. You'll never reach your fat loss goals by working out 1x a week.

• Jam out:

What helps me push through a workout is listening to my favorite music, so even when there's tough stuff ahead, it doesn't seem so hard when you're in your zone.

• Schedule it in:

Treat your workouts like an appointment. Schedule them in your phone or calendar, and block that time out. You have time for a 30 min workout or less. If you need to cut back on Facebook or TV, then do it. Those things will not help you get the perfect body for your wedding.

• Perfect form:

If you are performing an exercise with subpar form, then you're wasting time. The mission is to hit certain muscles, if you are not doing that, then you are not getting results, and you are wasting time. The better your form, the better your results, and you'll be less likely to get injured.

• Remember WHY:

Even the most dedicated will have difficult times throughout the 12 weeks, this is completely normal, just think back to your WHY. You need to remember why you started this, and why you will finish, because is quitting really an option?

• Pushing yourself: Intensity level

I won't be in your living room or at your gym standing over you making sure you are pushing yourself at every workout. But if you want this, then you better give it your all during these workouts, because what else are you going to save it for? If a certain exercise is for 30 seconds, try your all for those 30 seconds, if you need to take a few seconds break during the 30 seconds, you can, but make sure to get right back into the exercise. If you stop and rest when you know you shouldn't, you're only cheating yourself out of a better body.

This is your wedding! All eyes are going to be on you, it's the biggest party of your life, and YOU are the star of the party, YOU are in the spotlight, so let's do this right!

Know when to stop

While you want to get the most out of every workout, it's important to know when you should stop exercising and get help. If you are ever feeling light headed, in pain (other than muscle fatigue), or sick, then by all means take a breather and few minutes rest to recover, use common sense. **If you ever feel like there is something seriously wrong, stop exercising and if you need to, get proper medical help right away.**

The Exercises:

We've included pictures and instructions of the main workout exercises below so when you read the workouts, you'll know exactly what you're doing.

If you need more instruction, check out www.weddinggym.com/bookextras for more guidance.

The warm ups:

posture band hold

the move

- Using a resistance band attached to a door/something solid, stand with your feet shoulder width and grasp the handles of the band. Looking straight ahead, with your palms facing forward, pull your arms back so that they are by your side, held out a few inches from the side of your body. You do not need a lot of resistance on the band. Now drop your shoulders down, think the opposite of shrugging your shoulders up. Next, slide your shoulder blades together, opening up your chest at the same time. Now with the shoulders dropped, standing tall with shoulder blades sliding together, contract your abdominals so that you are not overarching in the lower back. Now hold that position.

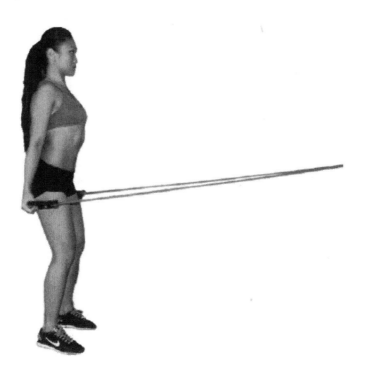

jumping jacks

start

- Start standing with arms by your side, feet together.

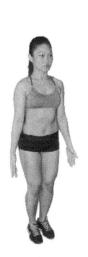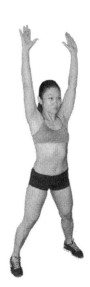

the move

- Jump your feet out to the sides while at the same time raising your arms out to the sides and up so that your hands end up above your head. Jump your feet together, lowering your arms at the same time to return. This is one rep. Repeat for reps or for time.

The main circuits exercises:

kettlebell swings

start

- Stand with your feet slightly wider than shoulder width. Look straight ahead and keep you spine in a neutral position. While keeping your shoulders pulled back, let the KB hang from your arms-your core braced.

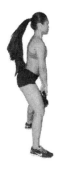 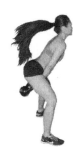 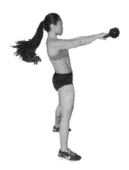

the move

* Push your butt behind you and then quickly push your hips forward, propelling the kettlebell up higher and higher each time you pop the hips back and forth. Aim to reach chin level with each swing.

mountain climbers

start

* Start in a push up position, hands placed below the shoulder, on the mat. Your legs are staggered, so that one knee is pulled closer to the arms.

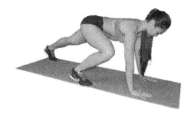 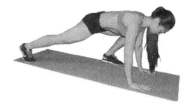

the move

- Your feet switch positions in one quick move, straightening out one leg, while pulling the other knee underneath you, pulling close to the chest. Keep switching back and forth for reps.

opposite knee mtn. climbers

start

- Start in a push up position, hands placed below the shoulder, on the mat. Same position as the mountain climber.

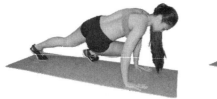 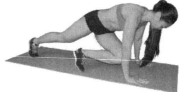

the move

- Your feet switch positions in one quick move, keeping the core braced, twist and pull your knee to the opposite elbow for each rep. Alternate back and forth quickly.

side lunges

start

- Standing with feet shoulder width apart.

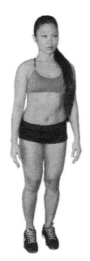 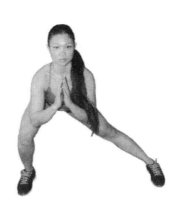

the move

- Step out to the side, shifting your weight to that outside leg. As you bend at the knee, push your butt backwards, as if you were sitting down. Aim to lower down so that your thigh is parallel with the floor. Straighten out the leg by pushing yourself back to the start standing position. Repeat on the other side.

single leg squats

start

- Balancing on one foot, place the other foot behind you on a chair, bench, or steps. Hold on to something if you need to while getting set up.

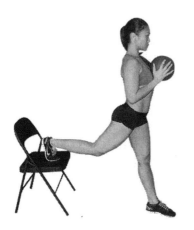 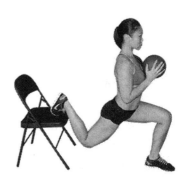

the move

- Drop the back knee down and backwards as you bend at the front knee, making sure that your knee does not forward past the toes on your front foot. Most of the weight should be balanced on the heel of the front foot. If it's not, position the foot even further forward. Drive up through the heel to come back up to the start position to complete 1 rep.

push-up hold

start

- Get into a push up position, with hands placed shoulder width, directly below the shoulders, on the mat. Raise the hips so that the back is flat and parallel with the floor. Imagine someone was going to punch you in the stomach, that's how you should be braced in the core.

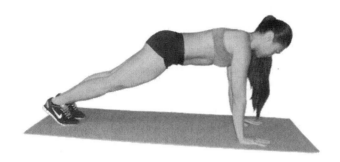

medicine ball squats

start

- Like any other squat, feet are positioned shoulder width apart. Hold the medicine ball in front of your chest.

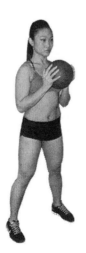
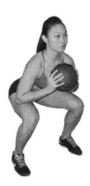

the move

- Holding the medicine ball, push your hips back, as if you were sitting on a chair behind you. Bend at the knees to lower yourself down so that your thighs are parallel with the floor. Your chest is facing forward the entire time. Your weight should be 75% centered on your heels as you drive back up, squeezing the glutes to stand back up.

band twists

start

- Set up a resistance band in a door, making sure that it is well secured. Hold the band out in front of you, so that there is no slack in the band.

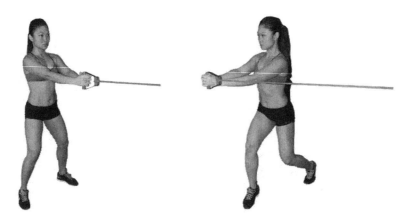

the move

- Keeping your arms straight and locked at the elbows, use your arms to twist to the side. Pivot on the feet as you turn, making sure to keep your core braced. Come back to the starting position so that your hands are back in front of your body. Adjust the resistance by moving further away or closer to the bands attachment.

wide squat jumps

start

* Squat down into a seated position, with your feet separated into a wide stance.

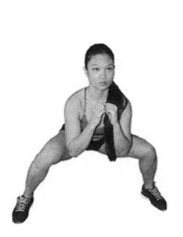 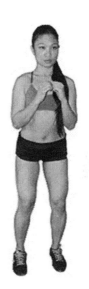

the move

* Jump up and as you come up, bring your feet together. Drop back down into a wide stance to restart and continue for reps.

resistance band rows

start

- With a staggered foot stance for balance, grasp the resistance band handles so that your arms are outstretched in front of you. Adjust your body closer or further away from the bands attachment point to decrease or increase resistance based on your skill levels.

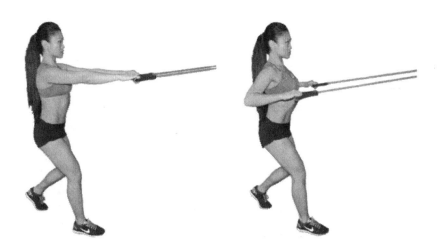

the move

- Think about pulling the elbows back while squeezing the shoulder blades together as you pull back on the band. Squeeze the shoulder blades and then return to that start position for 1 rep.

push-ups

start

- Place your hands shoulder width apart and below your shoulders. Your body should be braced and rigid, your hips should not be falling down.

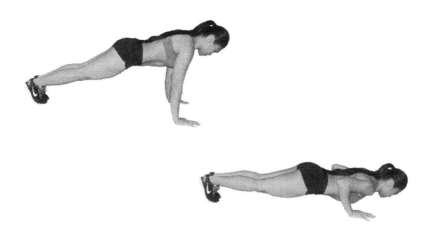

the move

- Brace your core and keep you elbows in close to your
  sides as you lower your body down. You should move as
  if your entire body was a plank of wood, straight and solid
  from head to toe. Once you reach the bottom position,
  push yourself back up into the start position. Imagine
  you are pushing through the floor with your hands. If you
  cannot perform a regular push up, drop to you knees, and
  keeping the body straight from the knees to the shoulder,
  perform the same way for repetitions.

seated knee-ins

start

- Sitting on the floor, place your hands down on the floor,
  slightly ahead of your butt. Raise your feet 1-2 inches off
  the floor.

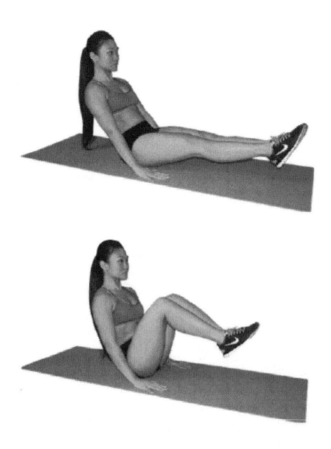

the move

- Keeping your feet together, pull your knees into your chest, squeezing your abs as you pull in. Straighten your feet back out, without letting them touch the floor. Avoid leaning too far back, as this takes the emphasis off of the abdominals.

oblique cross-over reach

start

- Lie on the floor with arms and legs outstretched into a X position, as if you were about to make a snow angel.

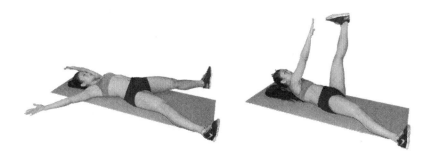

the move

- Lift up the left leg, while keeping it straight. Keeping the right arm straight, reach for the left foot so that the right shoulder comes up off the matt as you reach for the left foots' toes. Lower both leg and arm, and switch.

medicine ball thrusters

start

- Like any other squat, feet are positioned slightly wider than shoulder width apart. Hold the medicine ball in front of your chest.

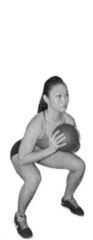
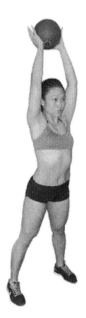

the move

- Squat down so that your thighs are parallel with the floor, then push through the heels to stand back up, pushing the medicine ball up over your head at the same time. You will come back down into a squat while lowering the medicine ball back to your chest and repeat back and forth. These are tough, but a great way to tone the entire body from head to toe.

jump squats

start

- Like any other squat, feet are positioned shoulder width apart. Raise the arms so that they are above your head.

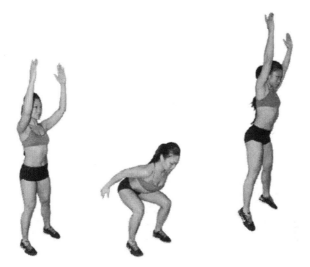

the move

- Swing the arms down fast and quick so that you come down into a squat position. Immediately swing your arms back up while jumping as high as you can. Land back down into the squat position and continue to perform reps, using the arm swing to help jump back up each time.

Finishers:

hip flexor stretch

start

- With one knee down, think about pushing your hips forward, while staying upright. You should feel this stretch on the front thigh and hip of the leg that is knee down. To get an even better stretch, raise the arm on the side of the body with the knee down. To get a real good stretch, make sure to push hard, if it's not uncomfortable, you're not doing it right.

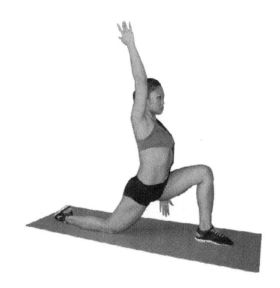

burpees

start

- Start out standing with feet slightly wider than shoulder width. Knees have a slight bend in them, and you are in a ready athletic stance.

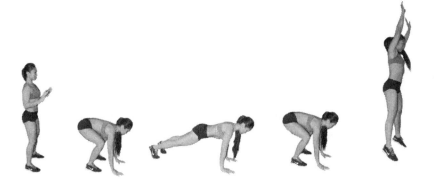

the move

- Come down and place your hands on the ground, now you will jump your feet out so that your entire body extends out straight, like you were about to do a push-up. From here, pull the feet back in to your chest quickly, and shift your weight back to your feet. Then jump up, swinging your arms up, as if you were doing a jump squat. Congrats, you've just done a burpee. Fun right!?

medicine ball jumping jacks

start

- In a wide stance, hold the medicine ball in front of your chest.

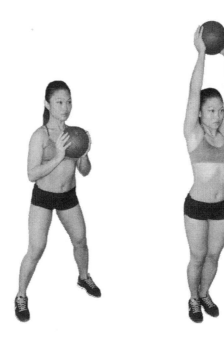

the move

- Jump up and bring your feet together like a jumping jack, while pressing the medicine ball straight up over your head. Jump your feet back out into a wide stance while at the same time bringing the medicine ball back down. Continue to go back and forth for reps.

Now lets move on to the workouts...

Weekly work out schedule
Phase 1
(Weeks 2-4)

Monday	Tuesday	Wednesday	Thursday	Friday	Saturday	Sunday
Day 1: Resistance Workout	Day 2: Cardio 30 Min	Day 3: Core & Conditioning	Day 4: Cardio 30 Min	Day 5: Resistance Workout	Day 6: Rest optional Cardio 30 min	Day 7: Rest

Monday — Resistance workout

Warm up 3x:	Reps/Time
Jump Rope	30 Seconds
Band Hold	60 Seconds

Circuit 1 4x:	
Kettlebell Swings	30 Seconds
Mountain Climbers	30 Seconds
Rest	30-45 Seconds

Circuit 2 4x:	Reps/Time
Side Lunges with overhead DB Press	30 Seconds
Push-up Hold	30 Seconds
Rest	30 Seconds

Finisher 1x	
Jumprope	2 Min. Non Stop

Tuesday — Cardio | 30 min

ie: Jogging, Biking, Rowing, etc.

for more ideas:
www.weddinggym.com/bookextras

Wednesday — (week 2) Core & Conditioning

Warm up 3x:	Reps/Time
Jumping Jacks	60 Seconds
Band Hold	60 Seconds

Circuit 1 | 3x: **Reps/Time**
Burpees   60 Seconds
Skaters   60 Seconds
Opposite Knee MC   60 Seconds
Rest   60 Seconds

Circuit 2 | 3x:
Power Jumping   60 Seconds
  Jacks
Plank to Push-ups   60 Seconds
Split Squats   60 Seconds
Rest   30-60 Sec.

Finisher | 1x   **Reps/Time**
Burpees   20 Reps
  (as fast as you can)
Hip Flexor Stretch   60 Sec. Each Leg

Wednesday (week 3) Core & Conditioning

Warm up | 3x: **Reps/Time**
Jumping Jacks   30 Seconds
Band Hold   60 Seconds

Circuit 1 | 3x: **Reps/Time**
High Knees   30 Seconds
Toe Taps   30 Seconds
High Knees   30 Seconds
Sholder Taps   30 Seconds
High Knees   30 Seconds
Seated Knee-ins   30 Seconds
High Knees   30 Seconds
Jump Twists   30 Seconds
High Knees   30 Seconds
Oblique Cross Over   30 Seconds
  Reaches
High Knees   30 Seconds
Rest   60 Seconds

Finisher | 1x
Side Plank, Plank,   4 Min Total.
  Side Plank   30 Sec. each position
                 (Move from right plank to plank to left
                 plank and then back to plank for 4 min.)

Wednesday (week 4) Core & Conditioning

Warm up | 3x: **Reps/Time**
Jump Rope   30 Seconds
Band Hold   60 Seconds

Circuit 1 | 1x: **Reps/Time**
15 Band Pulls &   5 Min Total.
  15 Jump Squats   (15 Pulls then wile holding the bands,
       go into jump squats, repeate for 5 min.)
Rest   60 Seconds

Circuit 2 | 4x: **Reps/Time**
Split Squats   30 Seconds
Plank to Push-ups   30 Seconds
Jump Twists   30 Seconds
Mountain Climbers   30 Seconds
Rest   30-45 Sec.

Circuit 3 | 2x:
MB Scoops   10-15 Reps
Diagonal MB   10-15 Reps
  Scoops (L-R)
Diagonal MB   10-15 Reps
  Scoops (R-L)
Rest   30-45 Sec.

Finisher | 1x
Skaters   2 Minutes
Sholder Taps   1 Minute
Jump Squats   30 Seconds

Thursday   Cardio | 30 min

Friday   Resistance workout

Warm up | 3x: **Reps/Time**
Jump Rope   30 Seconds
Band Hold   60 Seconds

Circuit 1 | 3x:
Medicine Ball Squats 30 Seconds
Band Twists   30 Sec. each side
Rest   30 Seconds

Circuit 2 | 3x: **Reps/Time**
Wide Squat Jumps   30 Seconds
Resistance Band   30 Seconds
  Rows
Push-ups   30 Seconds
Rest   30 Seconds

Finisher | 1x
Hip Flexor-Stretch   30 Sec. each leg

Weekly work out schedule
Phase 2
(Weeks 5-8)

Monday	Tuesday	Wednesday	Thursday	Friday	Saturday	Sunday
Day 1: Resistance Workout	Day 2: Cardio 30 Min	Day 3: Core & Conditioning	Day 4: Cardio 30 Min	Day 5: Resistance Workout	Day 6: Rest optional Cardio 30 min	Day 7: Rest

Monday — Resistance workout

Warm up 3x:	Reps/Time
Jump Rope	60 Seconds
Band Hold	60 Seconds

Circuit 1 4x:	
Kettlebell Swings	60 Seconds
Opposite Knee Mountain Climbers	60 Sec. each side
Rest	30 Seconds

Circuit 2 4x:	Reps/Time
Side Lunges with MB reach	45 Seconds
Oblique Cross Over	45 Seconds
Rest	30 Seconds

Finisher 1x	
Jump Rope	5 Min. Non Stop

Tuesday — Cardio | 30 min

ie: Jogging, Biking, Rowing, etc.

for more ideas:
www.weddinggym.com/bookextras

Wednesday — (week 5) Core & Conditioning

Warm up 3x:	Reps/Time
Jumping Jacks	60 Seconds
Band Hold	60 Seconds

Circuit 1 | 2x: Reps/Time

Jump Rope	60 Seconds
Push-up Hold	60 Seconds
Jump Rope	60 Seconds
Side Plank	30 Sec. each side
Jump Rope	60 Seconds
Seated Knee-ins	60 Seconds
Jump Rope	60 Seconds
Knee Jump-ins	60 Seconds
Jump Rope	60 Seconds
Rest	2 Min.

Finisher | 1x

Hip Flexor Stretch	1 Min. each leg

Wednesday (week 6) Core & Conditioning

Warm up | 3x: Reps/Time

Jumping Jacks	60 Seconds
Band Hold	60 Seconds

Circuit 1 | 3x: Reps/Time

Burpees	60 Seconds
Skaters	60 Seconds
Opposite Knee	60 Seconds
Mtn. Climbers	60 Seconds
Rest	60 Seconds

Circuit 2 | 3x:

Power Jumping Jacks	60 Seconds
Plank to Push-ups	60 Seconds
Split Squats	60 Seconds
Rest	30-60 Sec.

Finisher | 1x

Burpees (as fast as you can)	20 Reps
Hip Flexor Stretch	60 Sec. each leg

Wednesday (week 7) Core & Conditioning

Warm up | 3x: Reps/Time

Jump Rope	30 Seconds
Band Hold	60 Seconds

Circuit 1 3x:	Reps/Time
High Knees	30 Seconds
Toe Taps	30 Seconds
High Knees	30 Seconds
Sholder Taps	30 Seconds
High Knees	30 Seconds
Seated Knee-ins	30 Seconds
High Knees	30 Seconds
Jump Twists	30 Seconds
High Knees	30 Seconds
Oblique Cross Over Reaches	30Seconds
High Knees	30 Seconds
Rest	60 Seconds

Finisher 1x	Reps/Time
Side Plank, Plank, Side Plank	4 Min Total. 30 Sec. each position (Move from right plank to plank to left plank and then back to plank for 4 min.)

Wednesday (week 8) Core & Conditioning

Warm up 3x:	Reps/Time
Jumping Jacks	30 Seconds
Band Hold	60 Seconds

Circuit 1 1x:	
15 Band Pulls & 15 Jump Squats	5 Min. (15 pulls then wile holding the bands, go right into jump squats, back into pulls, etc for 5 min.)

Circuit 2 4x:	
Split Squats	30 Seconds
Plank to Push-up	30 Seconds
Jump Twists	30 Seconds
Mtn Climbers	30 Seconds
Rest	30-45 Sec.

Circuit 3 2x:	
MB Scoops	10-15 Reps
Diagonal MB Scoops (L-R)	10-15 Reps
Diagonal MB Scoops (R-L)	10-15 Reps
Rest	30-45 Sec.

Finisher | 1x   **Reps/Time**
Skaters   2 Minutes
Sholder Taps   1 Minute
Jump Squats   30 Seconds

Thursday   Cardio | 30 min

Friday   Resistance workout *(replace with test day on week 8)

Warm up | 3x: **Reps/Time**
Jumping Jacks   60 Seconds
Band Hold   60 Seconds

Circuit 1 | 3x:
MB or DB Thrusters   30 Seconds
Band Twists   30 Sec. each side
Rest   30 Seconds

Circuit 2 | 3x: **Reps/Time**
Single Leg Squats   30 Sec. each leg
Band Rows   30 Seconds
Push-ups   30 Seconds
Rest   30-45 Seconds

Finisher | 1x
Jump Rope   2 Minutes
Hip Flexor Stretch   1 Min. each leg

Weekly work out schedule
Phase 3
(Weeks 9-12)

Monday	Tuesday	Wednesday	Thursday	Friday	Saturday	Sunday
Day 1: Resistance Workout	Day 2: Cardio 30 Min	Day 3: Core & Conditioning	Day 4: Cardio 30 Min	Day 5: Resistance Workout	Day 6: Rest optional Cardio 30 min	Day 7: Rest

Monday | Resistance workout

Warm up	3x:	Reps/Time
Jump Rope	60 Seconds
Band Hold	60 Seconds

Circuit 1	4x:	
Kettlebell Swings	60 Seconds
Seated Knee ins	45 Seconds
Push-ups	45 Seconds
Rest	45 Seconds

Circuit 2	4x:	Reps/Time
Side Lunges with Overhead DB Press	60 Seconds
Opposite Knee Mtn. Climbers	60 Seconds
Rest	45-60 Seconds

Finisher	1x	
Medicine Ball Jumping Jacks	2 Min. Non Stop

Tuesday | Cardio | 30 min

ie:
Jogging, Biking, Rowing, etc.

for more ideas:
www.weddinggym.com/bookextras

Wednesday | (week 9) Core & Conditioning

Warm up	3x:	Reps/Time
Jumping Jacks	60 Seconds
Band Hold	60 Seconds

Circuit 1 | 2x: Reps/Time
Jump Rope   60 Seconds
Push-up Hold   60 Seconds
Jump Rope   60 Seconds
Side Plank   30 Sec. each side
Jump Rope   60 Seconds
Seated Knee-ins   60 Seconds
Jump Rope   60 Seconds
Knee Jump-ins   60 Seconds
Jump Rope   60 Seconds
Rest   2 Min.

Finisher | 1x
Hip Flexor Stretch   1 Min. each leg

Wednesday (week 10) Core & Conditioning

Warm up | 3x: Reps/Time
Jumping Jacks   60 Seconds
Band Hold   60 Seconds

Circuit 1 | 3x: Reps/Time
Burpees   60 Seconds
Skaters   60 Seconds
Opposite Knee   60 Seconds
Mtn. Climbers   60 Seconds
Rest   60 Seconds

Circuit 2 | 3x:
Power Jumping   60 Seconds
   Jacks
Plank to Push-ups   60 Seconds
Split Squats   60 Seconds
Rest   30-60 Sec.

Finisher | 1x
Burpees   20 Reps
   (as fast as you can)
Hip Flexor Stretch   60 Sec. each leg

Wednesday (week 11) Core & Conditioning

Warm up | 3x: Reps/Time
Jump Rope   30 Seconds
Band Hold   60 Seconds

Circuit 1 3x:	Reps/Time
High Knees	30 Seconds
Toe Taps	30 Seconds
High Knees	30 Seconds
Sholder Taps	30 Seconds
High Knees	30 Seconds
Seated Knee-ins	30 Seconds
High Knees	30 Seconds
Jump Twists	30 Seconds
High Knees	30 Seconds
Oblique Cross Over Reaches	30Seconds
High Knees	30 Seconds
Rest	60 Seconds

Finisher 1x	Reps/Time
Side Plank, Plank, Side Plank	4 Min Total. 30 Sec. each position (Move from right plank to plank to left plank and then back to plank for 4 min.)

Wednesday (week 12) Core & Conditioning

Warm up 3x:	Reps/Time
Jumping Jacks	30 Seconds
Band Hold	60 Seconds

Circuit 1 1x:	
15 Band Pulls & 15 Jump Squats	5 Min. (15 pulls then wile holding the bands, go right into jump squats, back into pulls, etc for 5 min.)

Circuit 2 4x:	
Split Squats	30 Seconds
Plank to Push-up	30 Seconds
Jump Twists	30 Seconds
Mtn Climbers	30 Seconds
Rest	30-45 Sec.

Circuit 3 2x:	
MB Scoops	10-15 Reps
Diagonal MB Scoops (L-R)	10-15 Reps
Diagonal MB Scoops (R-L)	10-15 Reps
Rest	30-45 Sec.

Finisher	1x	Reps/Time
Skaters	2 Minutes
Sholder Taps	1 Minute
Jump Squats	30 Seconds

Thursday Cardio | 30 min

Friday Resistance workout *(replace with test day on week 12)

Warm up	3x:	Reps/Time
Jumping Jacks	60 Seconds
Band Hold	60 Seconds

Circuit 1	3x:	
MB Thrusters	60 Seconds
Push-up Plank Hold	60 Seconds
Single Leg Squat with Over Press	30 Sec. each leg
Band Rows	60 Seconds
Jump Squats	60 Seconds
Push-ups	60 Seconds
Rest	1-2 Minutes

Finisher	1x	Reps/Time
Hip Flexor Stretch	1 Min. each leg

Workout Summary

- **Minimum 3 days a week:** Do the scheduled workouts Monday, Wednesday, and Friday (or other 3 day split like Tues/Thurs/Sat). For extra fat loss add in the cardio intervals for even greater results.

- **Save cardio for Tuesday and Thursday:** For an extra boost of fat burning, add some extra cardio in-between workout days. This means if you are working out Monday, Wednesday, and Friday, you will do running, biking, rowing, etc. on Tuesday and Thursdays. Keep it to 30 minutes. Short, but intense using interval type workouts.

- **Keep it intense and short:** No need to go past 30 minutes for resistance or cardio workouts.

- **Use resistance to get the most out of each workout:** Kettlebells will give you a full body calorie-crushing workout in no time. Embrace weights, and you'll see a slimmer and more toned you in no time.

- **Stay Consistent:** The *only* way to see results. You wouldn't brush your teeth once a week and expect to have clean, white, cavity free teeth…Get those 3 minimum workouts in EACH week.

- **Work out with a partner**: Recruit your maid of honor or bridesmaids, you'll have more fun, and get better results!

- **Make time to rest:** Make sure to rest one day in-between resistance workouts (you can do cardio on these days). Take at least 1 day per week to rest completely, meaning no exercise!

- **Make better posture a daily habit:** If you need to work on your posture, make sure to take 2-3 minutes out of the day to perform the posture band holds. With better posture you'll look younger, taller, and according to studies, even more attractive!

- **Have fun with it:** Make the workouts fun, play your favorite music and workout with friends so that it's something you will enjoy doing!

- **Make sure to record your results!** On test days, make sure to record your progress on the Assessment Sheet.

Chapter Four

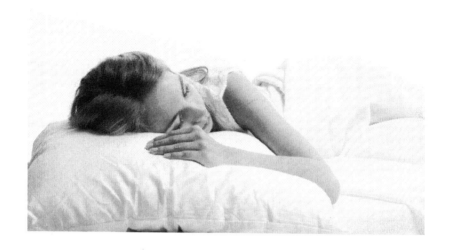

STEP 4: Recover & Reassess

For the final piece of the lean bridal body puzzle, we need to talk recovery and reassessment. In Step 3 you exercised and started sculpting the new leaner you, but during this process you are actually creating micro tears in the muscles. These micro tears can repair themselves to become stronger, leaner and more toned, by the recovery process. The recovery process is that time your body needs to transform. Without it, you will just continue to break down your body and become injured and weak, not sexy.

Rest and sleep are crucial parts of the recovery stage. Following up by reassessing your progress will ensure that you see the results you want and deserve!

Let's first talk about why rest is so important, and how to optimize it so you get the best results possible!

1) RECOVER:

Top 3 things needed for a slim & sexy new you:

1. Proper nutrition;

2. The right workouts; and...

3. **SLEEP.**

If you are not getting enough recovery, you could be destroying the physique you are working so hard for.

You regularly get 7-9 hours of uninterrupted sleep per night, right? In today's day and age, it seems like getting 6 hours of sleep is a luxury for most. Between work, workouts, and planning a wedding, who actually has time for more than that?

You do! And if you don't, you need to start planning it in to your daily schedule. Around 30% of Americans don't get enough sleep each night. What's crazy is that most people have enough time for sleep, but they just choose to stay up late. If you're trying to achieve a bridal bod by your wedding, you cannot afford to skip those ZZZs.

Sleep is when our bodies can repair all the damage we've done to it throughout the day and recharges us for the next. By skimping on sleep, you will interfere with muscle repair and toning process, possibly adding on the pounds.

Don't believe me? According to a 2004 study, people who sleep less than 6 hours a day were almost 30 percent more likely to become obese than those who slept 7-9 hours. And that's not the only thing sleep deprivation leads to.

What happens when you don't get enough sleep:

There's a reason, it's called getting your beauty sleep. There are many ways sleep deprivation can wreak havoc on your health, fat loss, and appearance!

- **You get OLDER looking skin:** Lack of sleep leads to an increase in the stress hormone cortisol, which affects collagen fibers, the connective tissue in your skin. This can lead to a greater appearance of lines and wrinkles and less elastic skin, which looks older than it actually is. (Interestingly enough, sex releases hormones that counteract cortisol's effects.)

- **You gain weight:** Lack of sleep results in appetite stimulation and affects the hormones that control appetite. This causes individuals to feel hungrier, but usually for processed and carbohydrate rich foods. If you've ever been up late, you'll know that you feel hungry enough to eat a decent amount, and many do. (There's even been the introduction of the "Fourth Meal" by Taco Bell. Great.)

If you are asleep, you can't feel hungry and can't eat, resulting in a slimmer you.

- **You become irritable and depressed:** Insomnia is usually the first symptom of depression. Those diagnosed with depression were more likely to get less than 6 hours of sleep, according to a 2005 national poll.

- **You will DIE earlier:** I don't mean to scare you, but a British study from 2007 that followed 10,000 civil workers found that those who got 5 hours or less of sleep, instead of at least 7, had basically doubled their risk of death from cardiovascular disease compared to those individuals who got 7 or more hours.

What 8 hours of sleep will do for you:

While many recommendations call for 7-9 hours of sleep, scientists say that 8 are ideal, as most humans naturally sleep for 8 hours when not kept up or woken up artificially.

The benefits are the opposite of the all the negative effects of sleep deprivation:

- **More Energy and Focus**

- **Better Looking Skin**

- **Slimming Down**

Ways you can optimize sleep:

- **Set a regular sleeping schedule:** Going to bed and waking up at the same time every day sets a schedule in our bodies so that falling asleep becomes easier.

- **Limit large meals and fluids 3 hours before you sleep:** Feeling too full can disrupt sleep, and drinking too many fluids can cause you to wake up in the middle of the night. While total time spent sleeping is important, the amount of continuous sleep is even more so.

- **Unplug:** This is one I have even been struggling with, but really does help. 60 minutes before you want to sleep, turn down the lights and start setting the mood for sleep. Avoid using computers, smart phones, or any other bright device. These electronic devices emit blue light, which actually mimics sunlight and keeps us more awake and alert. Once it starts to get dark, the body releases chemicals that start to initiate the sleep process.

- **Make the room DARK and QUIET:** Again, your bedroom should be very dark and quiet. I live in NYC and have street lights shining into my room if I didn't have my light blocking blinds there. Sleep is natural. Bright lit up cities and towns are not natural. You have to restore that natural sleep environment in order to optimize your sleep and health. If it's bright, get light blocking curtains, if it's noisy, sleep with earplugs or get a white noise machine (there are even apps you can download to provide cool white noise sounds).

- **Avoid watching TV in bed:** You need to condition your body that the bed is for sleeping and nothing else, otherwise you will have problems falling asleep in bed. Don't do work or watch TV in bed. If you need to do that, go into a different room. Or sit at a desk. Beds are for sleeping and other things, not for watching TV.

- **Make sure it's not overly warm:** The room should not be too warm. The body actually cools down to sleep optimally, and we all know that a hot summer night when the AC isn't working leads to a very cruddy night of sleep. It's better to be cooler than warmer.

- **Avoid intense exercise in the hours leading up to your bedtime:** Regular exercise has been shown to result in better quality sleep, but intense exercise results in activation of the sympathetic nervous system that can actually keep our body in an excited state, which is not what you want as your head hits the pillow. Avoid intense exercise within 3 hours of bedtime if you have trouble falling asleep.

- **Sex:** Not only a great workout, apparently sex can be a great way to help you fall asleep. Oxytocin is a hormone released during sex, which actually helps us calm down and fall asleep easier. It counters the stress hormone, cortisol that can keep you from falling asleep. So if you have trouble sleeping, getting intimate is a great (and fun) way to prepare for a good night's rest.

Sleep Summary

Aim for 8 hours of sleep each night. Schedule it in; your body will look all the leaner, healthier, and happier for it!

2) REASSESS:

Moving on to the second part of Step 2 is just as crucial to your fat loss success.

In Step 1, you assessed "physically", in terms of weight and body fat, as well as fitness level. Here you set goals that you wanted to achieve. Now that we've gone through the meal plans and workouts, we will be reassessing your progress and goals throughout the 12 week plan. Here we are talking about making sure to do the Test Days to reassess your fitness levels every 4 weeks, and to record your weight and take a picture of yourself WEEKLY.

Rules for Reassessing:

- **Stay consistent:** Remember that when reassessing each week with weight and pictures, you are taking them at the same day and time. Pick a time, say 7am Friday, and record the results.. Fluctuations in water levels throughout the day can throw off weight, if you take it at different times throughout the day. **Keep it Consistent!**

- **Be honest with yourself:** If you do not reassess where you are at, maybe you are afraid to step on the scale, and you don't want to look at the number, because perhaps you had a bad week and ate out more than you should or missed some of the workouts. By not looking at the numbers, you are only cheating yourself. You will still weigh the same amount, regardless if you check it or not. Don't bury your head in the sand. There's great courage in being honest with yourself, so go ahead and do it. Even if your numbers are not where you want them to be, don't be discouraged - get excited! You now have a new challenge to attack, and it will give you the motivation to come back twice as strong for the following week. Use this to power you through.

Just remember: **YOU ARE NOT YOUR WEIGHT.** That is just a number, and it will never define who you are as a person.

- **Reassess WEEKLY:** I know we said this, but just to make sure, I'll say it again. Taking weight and pictures each week will keep you accountable. You then have the flexibility to adjust if you are a little behind for any given week.

- **Every week is a new week:** Regardless of how well, or not so well, you did since the last assessment, once you finish the assessments, there will always be a brand new week ahead of you. It's a fresh start each week. So don't let road bumps or successes get to your head.

- **Getting great results? Don't party just yet:** I know many brides who start to get great results and start to celebrate, thinking they did so well, and they go out and eat whatever they want all weekend. The next week they are nowhere near their goals for the week, because their weekend of celebration totally threw away all the hard work from the week before. Be happy, but don't go crazy, channel that motivation into even harder work to keep those results continuing.

Chapter Five

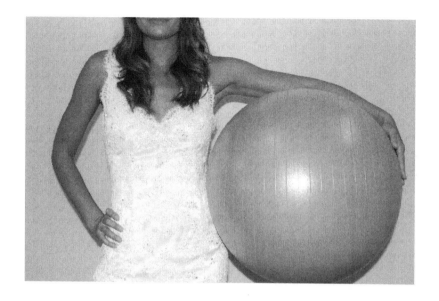

Fit For a Bride Summary:

Step 1: Assess for the Dress

Step 2: Eat Your Way Skinny

Step 3: Sculpt & Tone

Step 4: Recover & Reassess

These are the 4 steps that will lead to your new transformation, so let's just recap the most important points.

Step 1: Assess for the Dress (Week 1)

- Take your weight and picture. Repeat each week.

- Set your goals for where you want to be in 12 weeks.

- Complete initial fitness "Test Day" on Day 5 (Friday).

- Get all the things you'll need to get going! Fitness equipment and cooking supplies.

Step 2: Eat Your Way Skinny (Week 2-12)

- Alternating between higher and lower carb intake, based on what is indicated on meal plans.

- Eat more vegetables and avoid processed foods if you want to slim down.

- Eating lean proteins, healthy fats, and vegetables (fruits for breakfast) at every meal.

- Skip the calorie drinks and keep it to water and unsweetened green tea if you really want to burn fat.

- Stick to the meal plans and reward yourself each week with cheat meals.

Step 3: Sculpt & Tone (Week 2-12)

- 3 workouts each week will melt the fat and crush calories.

- Follow the workouts and push yourself to do more and more each time, that's the best way to keep getting results.

- To lose even more weight, increase the days of cardio.

- Keep working on posture every day!

Step 4: Recover & Reassess (Weeks 1-12)

- Rest completely at least 1 day each week - meaning no exercise.

- Optimize your sleep habits so you get 8 hours of sleep each night (no exceptions).

- Take weight and pictures EVERY Friday to make sure you are on track.

- Perform the Test Days on Day 30, 60, and 90 to measure your fitness progress!

Follow the meal plans and you'll be shedding fat. Use the workouts each week and you'll tone and sculpt. Recover and rest to allow the body to repair and refresh! Follow up with checking where you are and where you want to be. These are the steps I use with my bridal clients to get results like no other. It's a system that, if followed, will get you to your bridal body in no time!

(Caution: If you skip or neglect any part of the 4 Step plan, then you will most likely not get the results you want. It must be used in its entirety to be effective.)

I've gotten rid of all the guesswork and used years of trial and error, research and first-hand experience to create this system with all its specifics. Take advantage of everything here and use this guide to get your best body ever!

Chapter Six

BONUS CHAPTER:

Supercharging your fat loss

Next we'll go into what you can do to customize the *Fit For a Bride* plan for you. Maybe you want to lose weight faster, or perhaps you have lost too much and want to gain, or just maintain your weight. You'll discover how to use the workouts and meal plans to achieve your specific goals if you want more than just fat loss. We've also included the grocery lists, new recipes for fat melting meals, a guide to eating smart at restaurants, and a supercharged fat loss guide for those who really want to shed fat faster.

Customizing For Your Body Type

Customizing the plan for your goals!

While the meal plans and workouts are designed to work for almost everyone, some people have different goals than others, so there are a few ways to tweak the program to your goals. The way the meal plans and workouts are set up now, the results will be fat loss and total body toning. But what happens if you start losing too much weight? (Believe it or not, I have had this happen with clients.) Or what if you need to burn fat faster, because you have less than the 12 months?

I've had clients come to me and say, "Greg, I'm losing too much weight. I just want to maintain now". So we would adjust the meal plans and workouts accordingly. Below I'll show you how to adjust both aspects so you can lose more fat, maintain your body, or gain weight if you so desire.

Let's take a look at how to modify the meal plans and workouts for some of the most common goals among brides:

ACCELERATED FAT LOSS:

- **The Meal Plan Modification: Use Phase 3 (weeks 9-12) meal plans for all phases.** The time crunched bride, or the bride who has a lot more fat to lose before the wedding, will benefit greatly from adjusting the carb cycling in the meal plans. You will want to follow the meal plans from Weeks 9-12 for the entire time you have to lose the fat. It's more of a challenge to follow, but you will get faster results.

- **Workout Modification: Up the Cardio to 3-4 days per week.** Make sure to get in EVERY single scheduled workout and do 3-4 days of cardio, in addition to the scheduled workouts. The reason here is to burn more total calories each week. Since we already have 3 days of resistance training, the area we can modify is the additional cardio. Make sure to take at least 1 day each week to completely rest. You can do both a scheduled workout and cardio session on the same day if you want. Always do cardio AFTER a resistance workout, not before. You want your strength and energy for the resistance.

LOSE FAT & FULL BODY TONING:

- **The Meal Plan Modifications: None.** Follow the normal meal plans, and if you are losing more weight than you would like, replace one of the Lower Carb day's meals on the weekly meal plan with meals from a Higher Carb day.

- **Workout Modification: None.** Maintain the regular scheduled workouts with 2-3 cardio days each week

GAIN WEIGHT & PUT ON MORE MUSCLE:

- **The Meal Plan Modification: Replace Low Carb days with Higher Carb Days and add a snack.** You will want to eat more carbs on the Lower Carb days. By changing Lower Carb days into Higher Carb days, you will support more lean muscle growth and increase the overall body mass. This is ideal for women who are normally very petite and have a hard time keeping their weight up. An extra snack will add some more calories as well.

- **Workout Modification: Skip the Cardio.** Keep the cardio to a minimum. You want to keep the workouts mostly to the 3 scheduled resistance workouts. Avoid doing any excessive physical activity outside of the 3 scheduled workouts each week.

Use assessments to make adjustments: Because you are already measuring your weight and taking pictures every week, you are able to see changes to your body. Use this feedback to make adjustments when necessary. You might find that you reached your goals even before the 12 weeks is over, and at that point, you may want to just maintain your body weight and fat loss.

Fit For a Bride DO'S & DON'TS

I've had lots of clients whom were very successful in their bridal body transformation prior to their wedding. Here are some of their habits that got them and kept them skinny, sexy and healthy. If you are looking to tone and firm up, you might want to follow that success.

DOs

- Cook and prepare fresh foods for the week

- Grocery shopping at least 1x a week

- Incorporate resistance training

- Eat lots of vegetables. 5+ servings a day.

- Drink only water and unsweetened green tea

- Eat lean protein in every meal

- Eat healthy fats in every meal (olive oil, avocados, nuts)

- Minimum of 3 workouts each week

- Bring/pack food with you for healthy options at work

- Eat only when you are hungry, not because food is in front of you.

DON'TS

- Starving yourself: Load up on veggies and eat more veggies if you are still hungry!

- Eating processed "foods" (if its packaged it's probably no good).

- Eating fried foods, sugary things, and other foods you know are not part of the meal plans. (There's just wayyyy too many calories in these foods.)

- Giving up the foods you love. (Reward yourself with cheat meals weekly, in moderation.)

- Drinking calories. It's very easy to consume LOTS of calories while not feeling satisfied or full.

- Keeping "bad" foods around you at work or in your home. (If it's there, you will eat it.)

- Eating out at restaurants (Even the "healthiest" options at restaurants are not great).

- Making excuses. At the end of the day, it's an excuse. If you really want results, get it done.

- Skipping meals. Don't do it. You'll end up eating more (and then some) later. If you're hungry, EAT.

- Eating when you are NOT hungry. If your stomach is full, that food is going to be stored as fat.

Fat Loss Boosters:

Metabolism Boosters

The total amount of calories burned in a 24 hour period is known as the Total Energy Expenditure, or TEE. To increase fat loss, we need to increase the TEE, and one factor that affects that number is the process of metabolizing food, known as the thermogenic effect of food.

Certain foods and spices have a greater thermogenic effect, and by consuming these, you will actually increase your metabolic rate, burning more calories in a 24 hour period. I chose to include only things that research shows works, and this is what I recommend to my clients. I am about results, and that's what you'll get with these metabolism boosters!

Cinnamon and ginger are both natural and safe spices that can be added to smoothies, yogurts or protein shakes, and add not only a great flavor, but also have been shown to decrease body fat in studies. Green tea, caffeine, and hot peppers have all been shown to boost the metabolism for a few hours after consumption. So if you're looking for a low calorie metabolism boost, don't be afraid to add some Tabasco to your chicken or eggs!

- **Cinnamon**

- **Teas, especially green tea**

- **Caffeine**

- **Ginger**

- **Hot Peppers**

Supplements

I'm usually not a big fan of supplements. You should be able to get everything you need from the foods you eat - foods that nature has provided. With the entire supplement industry being pretty much unregulated (they are not considered "food" so the FDA doesn't regulate them), I rarely use or suggest any supplements to my clients. There are a few exceptions, however, which have shown to be effective with no side effects. Below are the few supplements that can add to your fat loss and leaner body, with the science to back it up!

(NOTE: While all of these supplements are considered to be safe, check with your doctor before taking any new supplement.)

* **CLA:**

Conjugated Linoleic Acid (CLA) is a naturally occurring fatty acid that can actually help you to lose fat. It's one of those healthy fats that are normally found in beef, butter, and cheese from grass fed cows, as well as from fish sources.

There have been studies showing fat loss just from supplementation with CLA alone, with no changes in diet or exercise. These subjects STILL lost body fat, not just weight, but actual fat. Now imagine adding a clean eating meal plan and super effective workouts? You'll be on your way to a leaner, sexier bridal body in no time.

Most studies used 3-6 grams/day, and as always, make sure you get an OK from your doctor before taking ANY supplement.

* **Fish Oil Pills:**

While I'm sure you've heard the benefits of fish oil pills, such as lowering your risk of stroke and heart disease, as well as helping with weight loss, the omega 3 fatty acids found in these oils can build a healthier you from the inside out. It helps protect your heart, joints, and leaves you with a leaner body on top of all that!

Studies have shown that just taking fish oil pills every day for 6 weeks led to fat loss of over 2 lbs., and an increase of 1 lb. of lean muscle. This means that individuals in the study did not change their diet or exercise, and still lost fat and increased their muscle just by taking fish pills each day!

Just like the CLA, imagine adding this to your super effective meal plans and body toning workouts? Holy moly.

In the study, subjects took 4 grams per day, so you should aim for 4-6 grams to see similar results. Each pill is about 1 gram usually, but always check on the label, and ask your doctor if they are safe for you.

One word of caution, you do want to aim for fish oil pills with the EPA and DHA in it. If you can, go for the refrigerated kind, and since pollutants have been found in larger fish, you want to get fish oils from smaller fish, like anchovies and sardines, it should say what fish on the label. Because these little guys are lower down on the food chain, they don't absorb as many of the pollutants that the bigger fishes are known to accumulate.

Diet

- **Cheat Meal Reductions:**

In the meal plans, I've set aside 2 cheat meals per week where you can eat any food you'd like; however, if you are looking to really slim down quick, replace one of those cheat meals with a low carb meal from the meal plans. This is a way to keep one cheat meal in there so you stay sane. I would advise against skipping the cheat meals altogether, just because if you do slip up, I've seen people then fall off the wagon completely for days. It's not good.

Extra Activity

Another major factor that can increase the total amount of calories you burn per day, is daily activity. So if you increase your daily activity (excluding exercise), you can supercharge your fat loss as you burn more and more calories each day. Those calories add up big time.

- **Stand more to burn more:**

According to the website, JustStand.Org, a 130 lb. woman would burn almost burn an additional 240 calories per day if she stood instead of sat for an 8 hour work day. **That equates to 25 pounds of weight loss in one year. Just by standing more!**

- **Getting outside and active:**

. Your body creates its own Vitamin D, but needs sunlight to do so! In addition to getting enough Vitamin D, the calming effects of reconnecting with nature can have a huge impact on your stress levels, which directly affect your weight loss efforts. When is the last time you walked barefoot outside?

- **Sexercise:**

According to Web MD, sex can have a serious extra calorie burning effect, which you can add on top of your regular workouts to get in shape for the wedding.

"Thirty minutes of sex burns 85 calories **or more**. It may not sound like much, but it adds up: Forty-two half-hour sessions will burn 3,570 calories, more than enough to lose a pound. Doubling up, you could drop that pound in 21 hour-long sessions."

Depending on how you do it, you can get a serious workout in here, both cardio and body weight based resistance.

Sex also releases certain hormones like testosterone, which can help you stay lean. It also leads to more DHEA which can also help fight depression, boost your immune system, and leave you with healthier skin…Who knew?!

At the end of the day, it won't be one thing or 2 things, but a combination of smart and healthy habits that will carve out your new bridal body and lead to a slimmer and healthier you!

Staying Lean While Eating Out: Surviving Restaurants

If you want to build a body that's wedding dress worthy, the one place you should not be frequenting is a restaurant. It is difficult to find appetizers and desserts at most restaurants under the 1000 calorie mark, and that's not even including the main course! On top of that, most portions at restaurants range from 2-3 times normal portion sizes and even "healthy" seeming options can have sodium levels through the roof!

This means you can easily consume more than 2 days worth of calories in just 1 meal! That's right, read it again: **2 DAYS worth of calories in just 1 MEAL!**

Once you realize this, you'll realize why most people with great physiques don't go out that often, and instead cook their own meals (which can be even more delicious than eating out at a restaurant).

When you head out, remember these 5 golden rules, and you'll be saving your hard earned body.

The 5 golden rules of eating out

1. Love the food that you're eating and don't eat it if it's not amazing!

If you are going to eat a cheat meal (which this will be) you better make darn sure that it's worth it. Make sure it's delicious, there's nothing worse than getting fat on calories that didn't warrant an Instagram post in the first place.

2. Skip the bread:

If the waitress/waiter brings out bread, just spit on them and tell them to get it out of your face. I'm kidding, but that's what you should be thinking. Instead tell them politely you don't need any bread. (REMEMBER: If it's there, you will eat it. If it's not there you can't eat it. You don't need to consume hundreds of calories even before your appetizer.)

3. Make it your cheat meal:

If you are going out to eat, make it one of your cheat meals. It's kind of a get out of jail free card, but the cheat meal rules still apply. You can eat any food you want, but not any amount of food. Keep portions reasonable. Which brings me to #4.

4. Split your meal or take half and have it wrapped:

Portion sizes are out of control. Split your meal with a friend or fiancé or have half of it wrapped to go before you have it served. (If it's there, you will eat it.)

This rule also applies to dessert. Split it! **Most desserts have upwards of 1000 calories each at popular chain restaurants.**

5. Order lean meat and LOTS OF VEGGIES:

I've yet to find a restaurant that doesn't serve vegetables. So when going out, look for meals that include grilled lean meats, chicken, pork, duck, or steak. Then load up on veggies. Avoid any meals that have "Crunchy", "Creamy", or "Cheesy" in them. This means major calorie overload.

Bonus Rule: Limit alcohol to 1-2 drinks & keep it to red wine:

Mixed drinks can have A LOT of added sugars, and we don't need to drink our calories, you'll be served more than enough on your plates. Alcohol inhibits willpower and regardless of what you're drinking, you'll be much more likely to go for that super chocolate chocolate cake if you've had more than a few drinks.

(While we're talking about drinks, unsweetened iced tea and water are your best bets, drink up.)

Stick to these rules when going out and you'll stay all the slimmer for it. Just remember that you shouldn't go out too often, but when you do, eat really great food, eat it slow, and enjoy it!

Kitchen Makeover Manual

Ok, so now that we know what foods we should be focusing on for a better body, we need to move onto the next step of getting rid of the foods we don't want to eat and getting the foods that we do need to eat.

There is a law that states: **"If you have something in your kitchen, you will eventually eat it."** It also works the other way: **"If you DON'T have something in your kitchen, you can't eat it."** This applies to both bad AND good foods.

We need to go through the pantries, the cabinets, and the fridge and literally throw out anything that might sabotage your bridal body transformation. If you have food at your desk at work, this is another area where you'll need to go through and replace lean body saboteurs with healthy slimming foods to keep you on track!

Step 1: Get rid of any "bad" foods

While I don't like using the term "bad food", there are foods that can trigger unhealthy eating, and you don't need that. Be honest with yourself. You know what should and should not be in your kitchen. If there are bagels or muffins you know you will eat, get rid of them. This can be hard for some people, but what's more important, eating that cookie or donut, or having everyone at your wedding tell you they can't believe how amazing you look?!

Are you serious about looking and feeling amazing in your dress on your big day? You are committed to getting results aren't you?

I thought you were, so let's go ahead and get going.

Pull out a garbage bag and remove all the boxed and packaged foods you have, anything artificial or sugary. Go through the fridge and get rid of anything artificial in there, anything processed, anything with preservatives, sodas, juices, leftovers, bread, and fake chemical dressings. The only things in there should be fruits, vegetables, eggs, milk, mustard, hot sauces, lean meats, and hummus.

But what about the foods I'm going to use for cheat meals? If you are only having one serving of ice cream or cake a week, you don't need to have a whole pint or a whole cake in your home. Go out and get an individual serving each week for your cheat meal. This will ensure you don't slip up!

Foods to get rid of:

* Anything processed: In a package or box.

* Breads, pastas, any "white" foods, white rice, bread, muffins, bagels, etc.

* Any calorie and carbonated drinks like soda, juices, beers

* Fake butter, fake salad dressings, and fake sauces

* "Low Fat" anything

* "Low Sugar" anything

* Anything that you know shouldn't be there

* Anything else that isn't natural

Step 2: Go shopping so that you have "good" foods.

At this point, you're thinking, well what the heck will I eat!! Take a look at the meal plans and you'll see the types of foods that you will be eating. All natural foods, like nuts, fruits, delicious meats, vegetables, cheeses, and carbs like brown rice and quinoa.

If you don't have the supplies for the healthy meals, then you can't eat healthy meals. If you don't consistently eat healthy meals, then you will not burn fat and tone up. You will get zero results. You want awesome results right? You want to look amazing when you put on that dress and walk down that aisle, right? Of course you do, so let's do it!

Below I've created grocery lists for you to use with each month's meal plans. You'll notice that the foods on the grocery lists are all natural, like fresh vegetables, red peppers, onions, broccoli, kale, and spinach. There are the super high quality protein sources to slim you down like chicken, grass fed beef, steak, and lamb. Delicious fruits and hearty nuts and seeds, all foods that are PACKED with nutrients and lots of stomach satisfying power, while offering fewer calories. Truly slimming superfoods that will be used to sculpt your body, and rebuild a healthier skinnier you!

Once you have cleaned out the kitchen, make sure to go out and get your slimming superfoods so that you are set to start cooking and prepping your weekly meals. It's a lot easier than it seems, and you'll save time and money at the same time!

Notes: You'll notice that for some of the foods, the amount is not listed. Some people will eat more almonds than others, and will have to buy more or less of certain foods. Same with nut butters, you usually won't have to buy a new container or peanut or almond butter each week, so just check how much you have and buy accordingly.

THESE ARE JUST GUIDELINES, the actual amounts you need to buy will be based on what and how much you are eating each week.

You do not need to buy everything on these lists if you are not eating those foods. Make sure you are only buying foods you need. Again, these are guidelines of the right things to buy. You do not need to buy every single item listed.

Grocery Lists

Phase 1: Weeks 2-4

Grocery List:

Lean Meats:

Ground Lamb 4 oz.
Chicken Breast, 1 lb.
Eggs, 1 dozen
Fish, 4 oz.

Nuts & Seeds:

Pumpkin Seeds
Raw Almonds
Almond butter

Dairy:

Low-Fat Plain Greek Yogurt
Feta Cheese
Goat Cheese
Low Fat Milk
Grated Parmesan Cheese

Vegetables & Fruits:

Broccoli Fresh or Frozen
Fresh baby Spinach, bag
Tomatoes
Bell Peppers
Kale, fresh or frozen
Yellow Onions
Chipotle Peppers, can
Blueberries, fresh or frozen
Mango Chunks, fresh or frozen
Strawberries, fresh or frozen
Limes, fresh
Avocados, fresh
Pears, fresh

Grains:

Brown Rice
Granola
Quinoa

Drinks:

Unsweetened Green Tea
Unsweetened Vanilla Almond Milk
Unsweetened Coconut Milk Beverage (NOT COCONUT MILK)

Condiments:

Extra Virgin Olive Oil
Hot Sauce
Cinnamon
Ginger, Fresh or ground
All Natural Vinaigrette
Hummus
Cracked Black Pepper

Phase 2: Weeks 5-8

Grocery List:

Lean Meats:

Grass Fed Ground Beef 4 oz.
Chicken Breast, 1 lb.
Eggs, 1 dozen
Wild White Fish, 4 oz.

Nuts & Seeds: (Buy in bulk and refill as needed)

Raw Cashews
Pumpkin Seeds
Raw Almonds
Almond butter
Shelled Raw Sunflower Seeds
Shelled Pumpkin Seeds
Chia Seeds

Dairy:

Low-Fat Plain Greek Yogurt, 1-2
Feta Cheese or Goat Cheese 2-3 oz.
Low Fat Cow's Milk, half gallon
Mozzarella Cheese, 1-2 oz.

Vegetables & Fruits:

Broccoli Fresh or Frozen,
Fresh baby Spinach, bag
Mixed Greens, bag
Fresh Arugula, bag
Tomatoes, 4
Bell Peppers, 2
Kale, fresh or frozen, bag

Yellow Onions, 2
Zucchini, 1
Chipotle Peppers, can
Blueberries, fresh or frozen, bag
Mango Chunks, fresh or frozen, bag
Strawberries, fresh or frozen, bag
Avocados, 1-2 fresh
Pears, 1 fresh
Orange, 2

Grains:

Brown Rice or Quinoa, 1 cup dry
Granola, 1-2 cups
Whole Wheat Pita, 2
Oatmeal, Old Fashioned 1-2 cups dry

Drinks:

Unsweetened Green Tea
Unsweetened Vanilla Almond Milk 1-2 quarts
Coconut Milk Beverage 1 quart (NOT COCONUT MILK)

Condiments: (Only get what you need)

Extra Virgin Olive Oil
Hot Sauce
Cinnamon, powdered
Vanilla Extract
All Natural Vinaigrette
Hummus
Cracked Black Pepper
Lemon Juice
Dijon Mustard

Phase 3: Weeks 9-12

Grocery List:

Lean Meats:

Flank or Skirt Steak Beef, 4oz.
Ground Lamb, Lean, 4 oz.
Chicken Breast, 1 lb.
Eggs, 1 dozen

Nuts & Seeds: (Buy in bulk and refill as needed)

Raw Walnuts
Raw Cashews
Pumpkin Seeds
Raw Almonds
Almond butter
Shelled Raw Sunflower Seeds
Shelled Pumpkin Seeds
Chia Seeds

Dairy:

Low-Fat Plain Greek Yogurt, 1-2
Feta Cheese or Goat Cheese 2-3 oz.
Grated Parmesan, 2 oz.

Vegetables & Fruits:

Broccoli Fresh or Frozen, bag
Fresh baby Spinach, bag
Mixed Greens, bag
Fresh Arugula, bag
Tomatoes, 2-4
Bell Peppers, 2
Kale, fresh or frozen, bag
Yellow Onions, 2

Red Onion, 1
Sweet Potato, 1 medium size
Blueberries, fresh or frozen, bag
Mango Chunks, fresh or frozen, bag
Raspberries, fresh or frozen, 1 pint
Avocados, 1-2 fresh
Pears, 1 fresh
Lime, 1

Legumes:

Pinto beans, 1 cup

Grains:

Brown Rice or Quinoa, 1 cup dry
Granola, 1-2 cups
Oatmeal, Old Fashioned 1-2 cups dry

Drinks:

Unsweetened Green Tea, (Loose Leaf)
Unsweetened Coconut Milk Beverage, 1-2 quarts (NOT COCO-NUT MILK)
Unsweetened Vanilla Almond Milk 1 quart

Condiments: (Only get what you need)

Extra Virgin Olive Oil
Hot Sauce, (Tabasco or other red pepper sauces)
Cinnamon, powdered
Vanilla Extract
All Natural Vinaigrette
Hummus
Lemon Juice
Cracked Black Pepper
BBQ Sauce

Chapter Seven

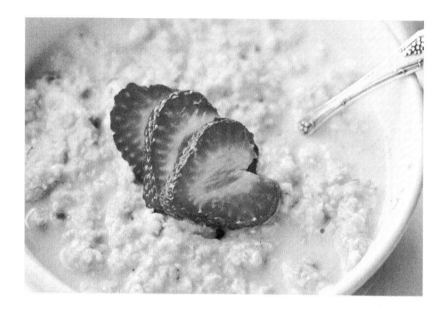

Quick & Easy Recipes: 5 Minute Meals

While there is lots of variety in the meal plans, it's always fun to try new meals and recipes. Here are some real quick, easy and delicious meals, along with some super healthy sauces to keep you satisfied and staying skinny!

Breakfast:

- **Spinach and Feta Omelet with Tomato**

Ingredients:

2 eggs
1 cup of spinach
2 tbsp. of feta cheese
1 ripe tomato

Preparation:

Heat a frying pan using a little bit of butter, then scramble eggs in a separate bowl. Add crumbles of feta and spinach to the eggs in the bowl, pour into the pan, cook both sides evenly, and then slice up uncooked tomato. Serve this on top of the eggs.

• Blueberry and Pumpkin Seed Greek Yogurt

Ingredients:

1 cup low fat plain Greek yogurt
1 cup of blueberries
¼ cup of pumpkin seeds

Preparation:

Add 1 cup of non-fat or 1-2% fat Greek yogurt to a bowl, adding in pumpkin seeds and blueberries on top. You can add a dash of cinnamon or a small drizzle of honey to add some extra sweetness.

• Strawberry Oatmeal with Flax Seeds

Ingredients:

1 cup cooked oatmeal
1 cup of chopped fresh or thawed strawberries
2 tbsp. of roasted whole or ground flax seeds
Dash of cinnamon (optional)
Drizzle of honey (optional)

Preparation:

Having precooked a batch of oatmeal, heat up one cup and then add in the remaining ingredients, with an optional dash of cinnamon, or drizzle of honey.

• Chocolate Peanut Butter Protein Smoothie

Ingredients:

1 cup skim milk
.5 cup water
1 scoop chocolate flavored whey protein
2 tbsp. raw peanut butter or raw almond butter
Dash of cinnamon (optional)
Optional 1/2 cup ice cubes

Preparation:

Combine all the ingredients in a blender until completely smooth, pour, and enjoy!

• Blueberry Pumpkin Superfoods Smoothie

Ingredients:

1 cup unsweetened almond milk
.5 cup water
1 cup of fresh or frozen blueberries
2-3 tbsp. shelled pumpkin seeds
.5 - 1 scoop protein powder
Dash of cinnamon

Preparation:

Combine all the ingredients in a blender and blend until completely smooth, pour, and enjoy!

Antioxidant Raspberry Smoothie

Ingredients:

1 cup green tea
.5 cups of milk
1 cup of fresh or frozen raspberries
1/4 cup of walnuts
1 tbsp. chia seeds
Dash of cinnamon
1 tsp. honey

Preparation:

Combine all the ingredients in a blender and blend until completely smooth, pour, and enjoy!

Skinny Pecan Apple Pie Smoothie

Ingredients:

1 whole apple, sliced (not peeled)
1 cup unsweetened almond milk
1/2 scoop vanilla whey protein powder
1/4 cup raw pecans
1 tsp. honey
Dash of cinnamon
Dash nutmeg

Preparation:

Combine all the ingredients in a blender and blend until completely smooth, pour and enjoy!

Lunch

* **Mixed Greens Salad with Citrus Chicken (Lower Carb Day)**

Ingredients:

1 chicken breast chopped
1 cup mixed greens (baby spinach, arugula)
½ cup sautéed vegetables
1 raw plum tomato (diced)
Lemon juice
2 tbsp. olive oil
Fresh black pepper

Preparation:

Adding the chicken, vegetables, tomato slices, and mixed greens together in a bowl. Drizzle the whole salad with lemon juice and 2 tablespoons of olive oil to finish off. Add ground black pepper to give a lemon peppery kick.

* **Quick Quinoa Salad (Higher Carb Day)**

Ingredients:

1 cup quinoa cooked
¼ cup sunflower seeds (hulled)
¼ cup diced onions
Sautéed peppers/vegetables
1 tbsp. olive oil
Optional: Tabasco and a sprinkle of parmesan cheese

Preparation:

Take the precooked quinoa, add in in the sunflower seeds, diced onions, and the vegetables you've already sautéed for the week, then drizzle in the olive oil and mix well. For an extra hot and cheesy bite, add in some Tabasco and sprinkle a bit of grated parmesan cheese on top to finish off. This can be eaten cold or heated up.

• Open-faced BBQ Chicken Sandwich (Higher Carb Day)

Ingredients:

1 grilled chicken breast
1 slice whole wheat bread
3-5 dill pickle slices
2 tbsp. BBQ Sauce
2 cups broccoli, steamed
Drizzle of olive oil

Preparation:

Heat up pre-cooked chicken breast, and toast whole wheat bread.

Top the bread with chicken breast and BBQ sauce. Top with pickle slices (optional). Serve with side of broccoli. Drizzle olive oil over broccoli. Add hot sauce for a spicy finish if you'd like!

To make it lower carb:

Remove bread.

• Strawberry-Spinach Salad (Lower Carb Day)

Ingredients:

2 cups fresh spinach
¼ cup red onions, sliced
½ cup quartered strawberries
2 tbsp. feta cheese
1/4 cup almonds, sliced and toasted
All natural red wine vinaigrette

1 tbsp. olive oil
Freshly ground pepper to taste

Preparation:

Dice up red onion and strawberries if they are not already cut into quarters. Combine all the onions, strawberries, feta, and toasted almonds into the spinach leaves. Drizzle red wine vinaigrette and olive oil on top, along with a sprinkle of pepper on top. Enjoy as a refreshing summer salad.

Avocado Lime Chicken with Rice (Higher Carb Day)

Ingredients:

1 grilled chicken breast
½ lime
½ avocado
½ cup pre-cooked brown rice (or quinoa)

Preparation:

Heat up pre-cooked chicken breast, or pre-heat frying pan with olive oil at medium-high heat, and then add a breast of chicken in a frying pan using some olive oil. Let it cook on both sides for 3-5 minutes until its fully cooked through, and is completely white with no more pink in the middle of the chicken.

Place chicken on plate, and add rice and sliced up avocado on top of the rice.

Cut the lime in half and squeeze juice on to rice and chicken breast. Use a sprinkle of salt and pepper on the chicken and enjoy!

To make it lower carb:

Replace rice with 1 tomato diced up, and 2 cups baby spinach or mixed greens.

Turkey Tomato Feta Salad (Lower Carb Day)

Ingredients:

5-6 slices of turkey breast
2 cups baby spinach or mixed greens
1 tbsp. feta cheese crumbles
½ cup cherry tomatoes
2 tbsp. olive oil
Cracked black pepper

Preparation:

Chop up turkey slices into small pieces and mix with spinach, feta, and tomatoes. Drizzle with olive oil and cracked black pepper.

Dinner

Tabasco Beef with Sautéed Onions & Peppers (Lower Carb)

Ingredients:

3 oz. of grass fed ground beef (Aim for 85% lean or higher)
½ cup sautéed onions and peppers
2 cup fresh baby spinach or kale
1 tbsp. olive oil
Tabasco sauce

Preparation:

Heat a frying pan and add the ground beef in small pieces, stirring so that the beef starts browning evenly. Add in the precooked sautéed onions and peppers, or if you have more time, you can cut them up and cook them with the beef. Keep the heat at medium-high, stirring everything around so that nothing burns. When the beef is fully browned, remove from the pan and add to the plate. Add fresh baby spinach to the plate and drizzle olive oil over the leaves. Add Tabasco to beef and onions to taste for a delicious and quick easy dinner.

• Balsamic Chicken & Broccoli with Chipotle Hummus (Higher Carb Day)

Ingredients:

    1 grilled chicken breast
    2 cups fresh or frozen broccoli florets
    1/3 cup chipotle hummus
    Balsamic vinaigrette

Preparation:

Heating up 1 grilled chicken breast, and either steam 1 cup of fresh broccoli, or if it's frozen, just follow the microwave instructions to heat up the broccoli. Serve on the plate with chicken and add the side of hummus. Drizzle the balsamic vinaigrette over the chicken breast and broccoli if you'd like as well. And voila you're done.

Making your own chipotle hummus:

You can buy premade chipotle hummus, or make your own real quick. Use plain hummus and buy a can of chipotle peppers in adobo sauce. You can add that sauce itself to the hummus and stir in, or use half a chipotle pepper with some sauce, adding into the hummus and stir well. Using more of the pepper will add much more spice. It's as easy as that!

• Fish with Sautéed Garlic Green Beans (Lower Carb Day)

Ingredients:

    3-4 oz. baked white fish or salmon
    2 cups green beans (frozen or fresh)

1-2 tbsp. olive oil
1 tsp. minced garlic
Fresh ground black pepper
Optional: Any low sodium hot sauce

Preparation:

Boil about 2-3 cups of water in a pot. Then heating up the pre-cooked fish in the frying pan with olive oil, add the minced garlic and black pepper to the olive oil in the pan. Once the water is boiling in the pot, add the green beans and keep covered for 5 minutes. Remove and add the beans to the frying pan, making sure to sauté the beans in the olive oil with the garlic and dash of black pepper for another 5 minutes. Remove the fish and green beans from the pan onto a plate and serve.

Add any hot sauce like Tabasco, or any other red hot pepper sauce for an additional kick.

- ### Cheesy Scrambled Eggs & Shallots with Mixed Vegetables (Lower Carb Day)

Ingredients:

2 eggs
1 small shallot peeled and chopped
1 oz. sharp cheddar cheese
2 cups mixed vegetables or broccoli (frozen)
Kerrygold butter

Preparation:

We're keeping this one pretty simple. Throw a cup of frozen vegetables in the microwave and heat up. Next, heat up a frying pan, and add some butter (Kerrygold if possible). You'll then chop up a small shallot, slicing pretty thin. Add the shallots to the pan, and stir around till they start browning. Then add in 2 eggs to the pan on top of the shallots and cook. Make sure to keep the heat medium to medium-high, as you don't want to burn the shallots. Flip over the eggs when ready

Serve the eggs on a plate and shave off 1 oz. of sharp cheddar cheese on top to melt. Serve with a side of mixed vegetables to make a super quick and easy meal.

Sweet and Spicy Honey Chicken (Higher Carb Day)

Ingredients:

    1 chicken breast
    2 tbsp. honey
    2 tbsp. olive oil
    1 teaspoon ground red pepper or hot sauce.
    1 cup mixed vegetables or broccoli (frozen)
    ½ cup brown rice or quinoa

Preparation:

Mix the honey, olive oil, and ground pepper or hot sauce together in bowl. Take chicken breast and coat it in the mixture. Cook in frying pan on med-high heat until fully cooked. Once you flip the chicken, add in the vegetables that have already been heated up (steamed or microwave) and cook altogether coating the vegetables as you stir them.

*DO NOT use the same sauce you dipped the raw chicken in on any other food. That's how you get food poisoning. Wash your hands after handling ANY raw poultry, including eggs.

To make low carb: Make 2 cups vegetables and remove the rice/quinoa.

Sauces & Dressings

• Fresh Avocado Vinaigrette

Ingredients:

1 avocado
1 tbsp. lime juice
3 tbsp. of olive oil
½ tsp. minced garlic
2 tbsp. white balsamic vinegar
Optional: ½ teaspoon of ground cumin

Preparation:

Combine all ingredients in blender and blend until they are all combined. Use on salads, chicken, fish, or pork!

• Skinny Bride Caesar Dressing

Ingredients:

½ cup 0% Greek yogurt
4 tbsp. extra-virgin olive oil
4 tbsp. Dijon mustard
2 tbsp. balsamic vinegar
2 tsp. lemon juice
1 garlic clove, peeled
Dash of salt and pepper

Preparation:

Add garlic, vinegar, olive oil, lemon juice, and mustard to blender. Blend until all ingredients are combined and smooth, then add yogurt and salt and pepper. Let sit in fridge for 1-2 hours before serving. **Serves 4**

Chipotle Vinaigrette

Ingredients:

2-3 tbsp. olive oil
1 tbsp. balsamic vinegar
1 tbsp. lemon juice
1 chipotle pepper
Dash of salt
Dash of pepper

Preparation:

Blend all ingredients together to make a delicious and healthy salad or sauce for chicken and steak!

Smokey Chipotle Garlic Sauce

Ingredients:

2 chipotle peppers with some adobo sauce from can
1 cup plain nonfat Greek yogurt
Juice from 1 lemon
1 tbsp. chopped shallots
½ small garlic clove, peeled

Preparation:

This one's another easy one, add in all peppers and sauce from can, then combine all other ingredients into blender and blend until fully pureed. Taste it when the sauce is a bright orange color, add a chipotle pepper, or some more lemon juice based on your preference.

A Special Message to You

Thanks!

For the bride reading this, I hope you have the most special day ever on your wedding and I hope I helped you on your journey. No matter what happens, you've got that special someone, and that's all that matters. Remember, they love you for you, the person they proposed to. So be happy!

I've spent half a year of my life creating this book, and if you take just a few of the lessons I've spelled out here, I'll be happy too. I'm very thankful that you've taken the time to read this book, it means a LOT to me, and I'm glad I could've shared it with you.

Need Extra Help?

While this is a pretty darn comprehensive book, as a book, it does have its limitations. That being said, I do offer an online interactive weight loss program that includes videos and actual coaching, so if that's something you think you may need, then don't hesitate to head over to www.weddinggym.com and check that out. Some people may find this book to be enough to help them; others may need more of the motivation and question answering when it comes to losing the weight.

Charity

Also, because we should all be doing good for others, 10% of the all book purchases go to St. Jude Children's Hospital, so it can continue to treat and save children with cancer without charging the families anything. I think that's a beautiful thing. As the founder of St. Jude said " No child should die in the dawn of life." I think we could all agree with that.

So thank you for helping with this amazing cause!

About the Author

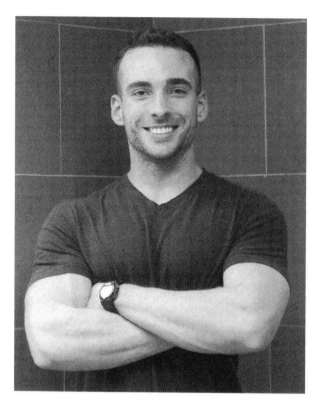

A Certified Personal Trainer by the American College of Sports Medicine, with a bachelor's degree in Health Behavior Science from the University of Delaware, Greg Doyle is a top personal trainer who works one-on-one with brides in NYC where he lives.

Since transforming his own body back in the 8th grade, Greg has continued to combine his love of food and fitness to change other people's lives.

Having worked with celebrities, world famous artists, and even royalty, Greg has found his passion working with brides, making sure they look damn good for their wedding. That's why he started The Wedding Gym. (you can check out his weekly tips and blogs over at www.WeddingGym.com)

He enjoys eating really good thai, and North Carolina style pulled pork. When he's not in NYC, you'll find him trail running through the Catskill mountains of NY. A redbone coonhound by the name of Ruger is his best bud, and they kinda love each other.

To reach him, you can email him at Greg@weddinggym.com, and he offers online interactive weight loss programs for brides who need extra motivation and expert coaching at the wedding gym website. www.weddinggym.com

Thanks:

Thanks To all the people that help made this book possible, all my brides out there, my great friends to name a few, Rich, George, Paul, Nicole, Meggan, thanks for making this happen. Thanks to Meaghan Shea, Brent Carter, Jason Dehenzel, and Michael Marasigan who are not only top notch trainers, but the mentors that got me started in professional training.

Thanks to my good friend Robert Bullock, the ridiculously talented designer and maker of gorgeous wedding gowns, who also provided a space and dresses for the shoot.

Big thanks to my Mom and Dad who have always supported me in my unconventional fitness career path. And thanks to God for making such a beautiful and special world that we all live in.

Credits & Acknowledgments

The information in this book is meant to supplement, not replace proper exercise training. All forms of exercise pose some inherent risks. The editors and author advise readers to take full responsibility for their safety and know their limits. Before practicing the exercises in this book, be sure that your equipment is well-maintained, and do not take risks beyond your level of experience, aptitude, training, and fitness. The exercise and dietary programs in this book are not intended as a substitute for any exercise routine or dietary regimen that may have been prescribed by your doctor. As with all exercise and dietary programs, you should get your doctors approval before beginning. Any mentions of specific companies, organizations, or authorities in this book do not imply endorsement by the author or publisher, nor does mention of specific companies, organizations, or authorities imply that they endorse this book, the author, or the publisher. Internet addresses and telephone numbers given in this book were accurate at the time it went to press.

© 2014 by The Wedding Gym, LLC

All rights reserved. No part of this publication may be reproduced or transmitted in any form or by any means, electronic or mechanical, including photocopying, recording, or any other information storage and retrieval system, without the written permission of the publisher.

Cover Design and Graphic Design by Meggan Arias

Editing by Kim Hayashida

Formatting and Layout by Jimmy Sevilleno

Project Manager: Rich Goldberg

Cover Photo by Paul Jochico

Dresses provided by Robert Bullock Bride - Bridal Collection in NYC

Modeling by Nicole Xenides & Maria Callanta

Getting Started Photo: ©iStockphoto.com/Freerick_K

Assess For the Dress Photo: ©iStockphoto.com/Kzenon

Meal Plans Photo: ©iStockphoto.com/Elena Gaak

Recipes Photo: ©iStockphoto.com/Stephanie Frey

Rest and Recovery Photo: ©iStockphoto.com/Fotek

Printed in Great Britain
by Amazon

26538173R00095